KU-530-039

Contents

Foreword

The study of ageing in all its aspects, both applied and theoretical, has until recently been a Cinderella subject – one of those areas considered worthy but rather dull. However, like Cinderella, the study of ageing has blossomed in recent years into something rather desirable, and at last it is receiving the attention it deserves.

Alas, a depressingly high percentage of this work has fallen foul of the old criticism of psychology – namely, that it tells us what we already know in words we don't understand. Picking a journal at random (which had better not be named), I find high-blown statistically complex articles that tell me that older people forget things more often than younger people; older people are considered intellectually weaker than younger adults; and family caregivers looking after a demented relative find the experience rather stressful and depressing. Of course, such papers are very erudite, have found new models for explaining the phenomena with slightly more statistical accuracy than the previous models, and I am sure they are all more than worth the grant money used to produce them. But often what is lacking is apparent contact with the everyday world. I can think of examples of test participants I have seen who, on conventional psychological tests in a laboratory setting, would pass with flying colours, but who sincerely believe that clouds are alive and that the quantity of clay changes when it is rolled out from a ball into a sausage shape. I also know from personal experience the delights of caring for demented relatives and have seen the immense dedication and patience shown by nurses in tending to demented patients (sometimes for their pains being patronised by unbelievably arrogant doctors, but that is another story). The sad truth is that much research either fails to make contact with reality, or shows one aspect of it, or trivialises the experience by being little more than a gloss of a complex issue.

That is why this book is a welcome relief. It provides a robust, common-sense approach to a complex but highly important set of themes. Those wanting a basic 'how to' guide will not be disappointed, but nor will readers who want to examine the theoretical underpinnings of a particular topic. I will not go through the rich and varied content of the book, because Helen Taylor does an excellent job of summarising this in the first chapter. However, I will note that the book escapes the alternative pitfall of becoming little more than a set of anecdotes without any theoretical or empirical rigour. The academic work is there aplenty, but it is made to serve real life experience, which in this instance is how it should be.

Beyond merely informing, the book should also provide a source of support (I would say 'empowerment' but the word has become horribly over used) to many practitioners reading it. We all have the capacity to make mistakes or feel anger or frustration at someone in our care. Reading this book should make one realise that, although there are boundaries that should never be crossed, one is not alone, and from that should come greater wisdom and understanding.

I hope that you will gain the same pleasure reading this book that I have done and will not only attain new insights but also carry these insights forward into your working lives.

Ian Stuart-Hamilton
Professor of Developmental Psychology
University of Glamorgan
July 2005

About the author

Helen Taylor is a registered nurse with experience of caring for older adults in a variety of care environments. She has a strong commitment to providing quality care for this patient group. She has recently completed PhD research investigating how nurses assess older adults in their care, and is now working as a Senior Lecturer in Adult Nursing at University College Worcester.

She is married with two sons and lives in Worcestershire.

Acknowledgements

This book is based on literature reviewed as part of a PhD research study jointly sponsored by University College Worcester and the Royal College of Nursing.

I would like to thank Dr Paul McDonald for all his help and support with the research.

This book is for Tom, Wil and Joe Taylor – my special people.

Chapter 1

Introduction

Setting the scene

There is much talk of the 'ageing population', and it is certainly true that for the first time ever there are more people aged over 60 years in the UK than there are below the age of 16 years.[1] The 2001 UK Census revealed that whereas 16% of the population was aged over 60 years on the 1951 Census Day, this had increased to 20% 50 years later. The proportion of those aged over 85 years also increased during this period, from 0.4% (0.2 million) to 1.9% (1.1 million).[1]

The primary aim of this book is to investigate the way in which nurses assess older adults who are in their care. By differentiating between this and other client groups, there is an implication that their needs differ in some way. Indeed, it is acknowledged that although not a homogenous group, older adults do form a special group, often with their own special requirements.[2] While it should be pointed out that many older adults live active and independent lives, free from illness and other incapacity, this is certainly not true for all. For these individuals, their continuing independence may be reliant on the input and support of healthcare professionals, including nurses. Indeed, statistics issued by Age Concern UK[3] indicate that in one three-month period during 2002, those aged over 75 years were almost twice as likely to have visited a hospital outpatients or emergency department as younger adults (25% compared with 14%). If an overnight hospital stay had been necessary, this would have been almost twice as long for the over-75s than for the younger age group (12 nights compared with seven nights). Older adults are also more likely to need some help and support with their daily living, requiring them to live in sheltered housing (19% of those aged over 85 years compared with 4% of 65–69 year olds), for example.

However, if the needs of an older person become too great and life at home is no longer an option, care in a care home or hospital may become necessary. This is usually because they are in need of a combination of medical, personal and nursing assistance.[4] The probability of becoming a long-term resident in a care home or hospital increases with age (20.7% of those aged over 85 years compared with 0.9% of 65–74 year olds). As such care commences, the patient will need to be assessed in order to identify and evaluate their needs,[5,6] and if nursing needs are identified, nurses will then work with that individual in an attempt to accommodate these needs.[7]

Davies *et al.*[8] conducted a review of the relevant literature and concluded that if patients are to be afforded a maximum level of independence and autonomy, their nursing care must accommodate their own particular and individual needs. It was proposed that effective assessment and subsequent individualised care planning are necessary components of this.[9] However, extensive research has been conducted into the nursing assessment of the older adult,[10–14] and issues have been raised relating to the reliability and validity of assessment practices.[15–17]

A number of concerns have been raised about how nurses actually conduct assessments. Middleton[18] has suggested that rather than promoting the collection of objective patient information, assessments may simply be used as a means of formatting and presenting the nurse's pre-made decisions. The criticism has also been made that the process of assessment is in itself restrictive, confining data collected to the format prescribed by the tool being used.[19] It has also been proposed that where nurses are required to select from predetermined assessment options, the option selected may not adequately represent the patient.[20,21] In addition, concerns have been voiced about the accuracy of assessments made by assessors who lack the skill or training necessary to complete those assessments.[6]

That being said, recent Department of Health publications have emphasised the importance of effective nursing assessment in the planning and delivery of care to the older adult, for quality assurance, to enable the 'costing' of the registered nursing care of older adults and to ensure consistency in the provision of care.[7] However, although the ethical, professional and legal significance of involving older patients in assessment of their health status and needs has been asserted, there is strong evidence that, for a variety of reasons, such collaboration may not occur. Other potential problems have also been raised, including a lack of consistency in the assessment of older people,[4] compounded by ineffective communication between care professionals.[22]

An overview of the book

It is clear that any deficits in the assessment process would have an impact on the reliability and validity of any evaluation of patient needs, and thus the care that the patients receive. The primary aim of this book is therefore to explore the way in which nurses assess the older adults in their care, and to identify and address potential problems and deficiencies with regard to the assessment process, both for individual patients and for older adults as a group.

The difficulties associated with establishing older adults as a distinct group have already been mentioned in this introduction. That being said, it cannot be denied that the healthcare needs of older adults do differ from those of younger adults,[4] or that a significant proportion of older adults do need some form of healthcare intervention. This is demonstrated by the fact that the NHS and social services spent approximately 40% and 50%, respectively, of their budgets on people aged over 65 years in the year 1998–99.[23] In addition to this, from 31 March 2001 there were 269 760 residential care home beds for older people in the UK.[24]

Much has already been said about assessment (for a definition of this concept, see p. 7). Having considered this, Chapter 2 explores the idea of old age itself, and gives an indication of the difficulties and potential dangers that are encountered when defining and classifying older adults as a group. Care needs specific to older adults are then identified. This chapter concludes with an overview of the political context of assessment, and identifies a number of key policy reforms in the provision of care for older adults.

Having examined the concept of assessment, and the special care needs of older adults, Chapter 3 explores the contribution of registered nurses to the care of older adults, and analyses this in relation to recent government publications and reforms. Furthermore, subsequent sections address the suggestion that individual patients and nurses may have different expectations of the registered nursing role. Difficulties associated with defining nursing needs are then appraised.

Further to considering the professional and political role of nurses in the assessment and provision of care for older adults, Chapter 4 looks at the process of assessment itself. Judgement and decisions are established as being inherent to the assessment process, with three different perspectives of decision-making theory being evaluated, namely information processing, intuition and the cognitive continuum. Having considered the decision-making process, the need for decisions to be reliable and valid is deliberated, and finally the issue of accuracy in decision making is explored and defined.

While Chapter 4 was concerned with the cognitive processes associated with decision making and assessment, Chapter 5 goes on to provide an overview of a number of ways in which the nurse who is making the assessment may compromise its reliability and validity. For example, the role of memory and information recall are explored. The possibility that the way in which a nurse regards their patients could influence the reliability and validity of an assessment is also considered.

Having explored the role of the nurse in the assessment process, Chapter 6 investigates the many and complex ways in which the nurse, the patient and other healthcare professionals interact during the assessment process. The areas considered include older adults' expectations of healthcare services, the role of informal caregivers, and the effect of culture and taboos. Some additional ways in which the efficacy of the assessment process may be compromised are also highlighted.

The book concludes with an evaluation of the ethical, professional and legal implications of assessing older adults. The emphasis is placed firmly on both the need and the requirement for the patient to be involved in assessment and decision making. This is considered in relation both to ethical theories and principles, and to professional obligations, including those imposed by the Nursing and Midwifery Council. There is also a strong legal impetus for nurses to involve their patients in decisions relating to their care, and a number of relevant issues are considered, including consent, confidentiality, Do Not Attempt Resuscitation orders and the Human Rights Act (1998).

The author's perspective

At this point I would like to reiterate that in no way do I wish old age to be regarded as synonymous with frailty and dependence. However, I am very aware that, for some older adults, advanced age does bring with it the need for help (to varying degrees) from healthcare professionals.

In my capacity as a relative, a nurse and an academic I have witnessed much very good care where nurses and other healthcare professionals have fully respected the autonomy and individuality of their older patients. These people have worked in partnership with the patient, and acknowledged their right to privacy, respect and dignity. I recognise that such an approach to care is often not easy, but have stated elsewhere[25,26] just how important I think it is for us to recognise the human needs of our patients.

Sadly, there have been occasions when I have either witnessed or myself delivered care that has fallen short of this standard, and this has always been deeply upsetting for me. There have been cases where the patient has not been valued as a true fellow human being, and their wishes have been either ignored or not sought. There have also been situations where the patient's dignity has not been preserved, and they have not been treated with respect. For example, patients with cognitive impairment (and even those without such impairment) may not have been fully involved in the selection of their meals and clothing, or may not have been given a true opportunity to decide how they would like to spend their day. These are some quite fundamental decisions and something that most of us would take for granted. Indeed, we have a moral and legal right to make these decisions, and we have the facility to seek legal redress should these rights be infringed. Just imagine for a moment how it would feel to be Miss Perkins.

Miss D H Perkins

I am not one for company,
and being on display all arranged in a neat semicircle
around the TV to while the hours away.
I hate that old Irish eejit and those noisy 'sing-a-longs'.
I just long to be alone in my room
With my radio on.
I want to feel fresh wind in my face
And not be surrounded by the stench of impending death.
Oh how my stomach churns
At the sight of spittle and pee.
I am not supposed to notice,
You think I cannot see.
Well actually yes, I can.
And I can certainly hear
All those things that you gossip about,
When you are making my bed . . .
Or feeding me breakfast . . .
Or combing my hair . . .
Oh, here you are now,
'Come on now Dottie,
It's time for your bath,
And then I'll get you a nice cup of tea.'
Well, I don't want a bath
And I don't even like tea.
And I hate lying exposed
While your eyes mock me.
I can see what you are thinking . . .
'If I ever get like that, I'll . . .'
Trust me you will, and no, you won't.
You'll just get on with it,
Like I do, day after day.
Month after endless month.

All you'll have is thinking,
Maybe not even that.
But I certainly do,
And in this gnarled old shell,
I know what I know.
That I hate mashed potato,
And wearing this dress.
That my leg is sore and aching,
And my hair is a mess.
I just want someone to listen,
Someone to see,
That I am still a person,
That I am still me,
And that to you lot I am Miss Perkins,
And not plain 'Dottie'.

H J Taylor

As a registered nurse I know that when care is below standard, excuses can be made – 'I didn't have enough time', 'we are so understaffed' or 'I just didn't realise . . .'. However, I believe that these are not sufficient reason to treat our older patients in ways that we would not want our parents, our grandparents or ourselves to be treated. I can do little about the first two excuses, but hope that this book will help to obviate the third.

References

1 National Statistics (2004) *Census 2001: population data*; www.statistics.gov.uk/census2001/demographic_uk.asp (accessed 03/04/04).
2 Stuart-Hamilton I (2000) *The Psychology of Ageing: an introduction* (3e). Jessica Kingsley Publishers, London.
3 Age Concern (2005) *Some Basic Facts 2004. Older people in the United Kingdom: health and social care services*; www.ageconcern.org.uk/AgeConcern/information_2662.htm#-Health (accessed 21/02/05).
4 Department of Health (2001) *National Service Framework for Older People*. Department of Health, London.
5 Heath H (2000) Assessing older people. *Elderly Care*. **11**: 27–8.
6 Richardson J (2001) The easy-care assessment system and its appropriateness for older people. *Nursing Older People*. **13**: 17–19.
7 Department of Health (2001) *NHS-Funded Nursing Care. Practice guide and workbook*. Department of Health, London.
8 Davies S, Laker S and Ellis L (1997) Promoting autonomy and independence for older people within nursing practice: a literature review. *J Adv Nurs*. **26**: 408–17.
9 Challis D *et al.* (2004) The value of specialist clinical assessment of older people prior to entry to care homes. *Age Ageing*. **33**: 25–34.
10 Ford P and McCormack B (1999) Determining older people's need for registered nursing in continuing healthcare: the contribution of the Royal College of Nursing's Older People Assessment Tool. *J Clin Nurs*. **8**: 731–42.
11 Fries BE *et al.* (2001) Pain in US nursing homes: validating a pain scale for the minimum data set. *Gerontologist*. **41**: 173–9.
12 Morris JN *et al.* (1990) Designing the National Resident Assessment Instrument for nursing homes. *Gerontologist*. **30**: 293–307.

13 Phillips CD *et al.* (1997) Association of the Resident Assessment Instrument (RAI) with changes in function, cognition and psychosocial status. *J Am Geriatr Soc.* **45:** 986–93.
14 Valk M *et al.* (2001) Measuring disability in nursing home residents: validity and reliability of a newly developed instrument. *J Gerontol B Psychol Sci Soc Sci.* **56:** 187–91.
15 Heath H (2000) The nurse's role in assessing an older person. *Elderly Care.* **12:** 23–4.
16 Philp I and Dunleavy J (1994) Community health assessment of elderly people: the national picture. *Health Soc Care Commun.* **12:** 117–19.
17 Gallinagh R, Slevin E and McCormack B (2000) Side rails as physical restraints: the need for appropriate assessment. *Nursing Older People.* **13:** 20–25.
18 Middleton L (1994) Little boxes are not enough. *Care Weekly.* **20 January** (cited in Nolan M and Caldock K (1996) Assessment: identifying the barriers to good practice. *Health Soc Care Commun.* **4:** 77–85).
19 Baldwin S and Woods PA (1994) Case management and needs assessment: some issues of concern for the caring professions. *J Ment Health.* **3:** 311–22.
20 Taylor H (2004) *The nursing assessment of older adults.* Conference proceedings of the Royal College of Nursing International Nursing Research Conference, 24 March, University of Cambridge, Cambridge.
21 Taylor H (2005) *The nursing assessment of older adults.* PhD thesis (unpublished), University College Worcester.
22 Reed J and Morgan D (1999) Discharging older people from hospital to care homes: implication for nursing. *J Adv Nurs.* **29:** 819–25.
23 Department of Health (2000) *The NHS Plan: a plan for investment, a plan for reform.* The Stationery Office, London.
24 National Statistics (2004) *Places Available in Residential Care Homes: by type of care home, at 31 March 2001. Regional Trends 37;* www.statistics.gov.uk/StatBase/Expodata/ spreadsheets/D5947.xls
25 Taylor HJ (2001) Patients have a right to respect. *Nursing Times.* **97:** 19.
26 Taylor HJ (2000) A caring moment with Margaret. In: A Ghaye and S Lillyman (eds) *Caring Moments: the discourse of reflective practice.* Quay Books, Dinton.

Chapter 2

The assessment of older adults: an overview

What is assessment?

Much reference has already been made in this book to the term 'assessment', but what *is* an assessment? One definition is that assessment is an instrumental part of the nursing process, whereby nursing problems are identified and a mutual effort is made by the nurse and the patient to either rectify or accommodate these problems.[1] Aggleton and Chalmers[2] define assessment as:

> More often than not a multistage process in which initial ideas are formed about existing health problems, followed by efforts to confirm the existence of these problems and to identify their probable cause.
>
> (p. 15)

However, Roper *et al.*[3] prefer the term 'assessing' to 'assessment' – to imply the need for evaluation of an individual's status to be ongoing, rather than a 'one-off' procedure. By assessing the patient, the nurse would then be able to place them on the continuum between dependence and independence for activities of daily living, and therefore identify any need for nursing intervention. In addition, Heath[4] emphasises the collaborative nature of assessment by suggesting that:

> Experiencing the process of assessment with an older person is an opportunity to learn more about the individual, his or her current situation, experiences, perspectives and desires for the future.
>
> (p. 27)

The convention appears to be that the term 'assessment' applies to a generic process, with a prefix defining the type of assessment. For example, community health assessment is an evaluation of an individual's need for community services,[5] medical and social assessments permit an evaluation of medical and social needs, respectively,[6] and nursing assessment is used to give an indication of a requirement for nursing care.[7]

Assessment tools

The Department of Health[8] defines an *assessment tool* as 'a collection of scales, questions and other information, to provide a rounded picture of an individual's needs and related circumstances' (p. 2). Assessment tools may be designed specifically for use by one group of professionals. For example, the Royal College of Nursing Assessment Tool for Nursing Older People[1] was specifically designed for use by nurses. The Minimum Data Set – Resident Assessment Instrument was intended for use by nurses and also 'experienced home staff under supervision'[8] (p. 11). However, the Camberwell Assessment for the Needs of the Elderly (CANE), the Functional Assessment of the Care Environment (FACE),[8] and EASY-Care 2002–2005 were assessment tools intended for multi-disciplinary use.[8]

A nursing assessment therefore involves the nurse identifying a patient's nursing care needs as a means of determining that patient's need for nursing interventions, and is part of the process of delivering individualised care. This assessment may be holistic and address the individual's biological, psychological and sociological health status, or it may concentrate on specific areas of need, such as cognitive status. Examples of tools used for holistic assessment include EASY-Care 2002–2005, CANE, the Minimum Data Set for Home Care (MDS Home Care), FACE, and the Royal College of Nursing Assessment Tool For Nursing Older People.[1] An example of an assessment that focuses on specific areas of health would be the Mini-Mental State Examination (MMSE).[9]

It is beyond the scope of this book to evaluate each of the many assessment tools that are available. This is because tools vary in their format, application and intended use, and a tool that may be of use in one particular set of circumstances may be less appropriate in another. In addition, tools are often updated on a regular basis by their developers, and may become outdated relatively quickly. However, the Department of Health does have information about a number of tools and scales which they have identified as potentially useful as part of the Single Assessment Process (SAP) (*see* p. 19 for further information on the SAP), and this may be a good starting point for readers who want to explore this further. Information about individual tools, and contact details for the companies responsible for their development, may be downloaded by accessing the following website: www.dh.gov.uk/PublicationsAndStatistics/Publications/PublicationsPolicyAnd Guidance/PublicationsPolicyAndGuidanceArticle/fs/en?CONTENT_ID =4005707&chk=bpfioP

Some examples of how assessment tools are constructed

'Open' assessments

These usually involve the nurse making a descriptive record in prose of their patient's status/needs. They may complete an assessment pro forma based on a model of nursing care such as the activities of daily living of Roper *et al.*,[3] or they may simply make an *ad hoc* entry in the patient's notes.

An example of the former approach is given in Box 2.1.

Box 2.1 Eating and drinking

Mr Smith has a mild weakness on his left side following a cerebrovascular accident last year. He therefore requires some assistance with cutting meat and other hard foods. He does not require plate guards or adapted cutlery, and he has no problems with swallowing. His appetite is generally good, but does tend to fluctuate from day to day. He reports that this is usual for him,

---

and that he prefers to be guided by his appetite rather than eat for the sake of it. Mr Smith has a preference for what he describes as 'plain foods' – he does not like spicy foods and never eats dessert. He likes to have frequent drinks (he will ask on an almost hourly basis if not offered) of tea (no sugar, just milk) from a china mug, and does not like coffee.

It is clear that presenting an assessment in such a way will enable the nurse to record many details of the patient's specific needs and preferences that would simply not be possible with some of the more structured assessment tools. Reading this assessment will provide other nurses with a reasonably clear idea of Mr Smith's eating and drinking habits. However, a number of the advantages and disadvantages outlined in Table 2.1 for 'informal assessments' would also apply here. For example, if the nurse was inexperienced, too busy or otherwise unable to make a more detailed record (*see* p. 63 for further information on inhibitors to effective communication), the entry could be much less informative (*see* Box 2.2).

Box 2.2 Eating and drinking

Mr Smith had a CVA last year and needs his meat cutting. He has no other problems with eating and drinking and enjoys a normal diet.

However, it must be said that even a response as brief as this will not have been suggested to the nurse, and therefore may be more relevant and accurate than some of those given when using structured assessment tools (*see* pp. 55–6 for further information relating to 'suggestibility'). Unfortunately, with both types of assessment nurses may opt not to make any response at all, and may leave a section blank, perhaps planning to return to that section at a later date. This will mean that in the worst-case scenario (*see* Box 2.3), no information relating to that patient will be provided at all.

Box 2.3 Eating and drinking

N/A

Some structured assessment tools also include open sections such as these to enable the nurse to add additional descriptive patient information.

Some 'simple' scales

As already stated, assessment tools come in a variety of formats, but usually the assessor will be provided with a number of options describing patient status/ ability. They will then select the option that most appropriately describes their patient. One of the simpler assessment tool formats is the visual analogue scale, often used in pain measurement (*see* p. 88 for further information on pain assessment in older adults). This will consist of a line extending between two points as follows:

Pain absent – – – – – – – – – – – – – – – – Worst pain imaginable

The patient is asked to rate their pain by making a cross on the line at the appropriate point.

Example 1:
Pain absent – X – – – – – – – – – – – – – – – – Worst pain imaginable

Example 2:
Pain absent – – – – – – – – – – – – – – – – – X– Worst pain imaginable

Example 3:
Pain absent – – – – – – – – – –X – – – – – – – – –– Worst pain imaginable

In Example 1, the patient has reported 'minimal' pain, whereas in Example 2 the patient would be expressing 'very significant' pain. In Example 3 the patient considered their pain to be neither 'the worst pain imaginable' nor to be 'absent'. Although this does appear to be a simple tool to use, there are a number of concerns relating to the reliability and validity of this method of pain measurement, including the following.

1 How do we know that patients have correctly understood how to use the tool?
2 How do we know that all patients evaluate severe pain in the same way? Some people could rate as 'severe' what others might regard as quite minor pain, and vice versa.
3 It would be difficult to compare the patient's evaluation of pain on one day with their evaluation on the next.
4 How does one evaluate pain that is rated around the midpoint? What is 'medium' or 'moderate' pain?

Other variations of pain evaluation scales might ask a patient to rate their pain on a scale of 0–10, sometimes known as a *pain thermometer*. Again, patients are required to rate their pain on the basis of descriptors – for example, ranging from '0 – I am experiencing no pain' to '10 – I am experiencing the worst pain imaginable'. Although this might give a more easily comparable measure (i.e. a number), many of the same concerns as those relating to the visual analogue scale will apply.

More complex tools

An example of a more complex assessment tool is the Barthel Index.[10,11] This requires the assessor to rate a patient on a number of items relating to their ability to perform specified activities of daily living, including feeding, bathing, dressing and bladder and bowel control. The scores for each item are then added and a total score is calculated, the maximum possible score being 100. A score of around zero would indicate that the patient is highly dependent, whereas a score of around 100 would indicate that the patient was largely independent.

An example is given in Box 2.4.[10,11]

> **Box 2.4 Toilet use**
>
> 0 – Dependent
> 5 – Needs some help, but can manage some things alone
> 10 – Independent (can get on and off, dress, wipe independently)

There are a number of benefits associated with using a tool such as this (*see* Table 2.1). They include the following.

1   A framework for assessment is provided to guide the nurse.
2   Calculation of an 'assessment score' could enable the nurse to make a comparison of that patient's need/status with the scores obtained for other patients, or for the same patient at another time.
3   Amalgamation of assessment scores would allow evaluation of general levels of patient dependency on a particular ward or unit.

However, the use of this scale again raises a number of concerns.

1   The scale measures what the patient actually *does* rather than what they are able to do.[12] Someone may be *able* to access the toilet independently, but for a variety of reasons (patient attitude, mood, enforced dependency by nurses/ other carers, environmental problems, etc.) may not do so.
2   It may be difficult to differentiate between *needing some help* and being *dependent*. These descriptors are open to interpretation. For example, how does one evaluate when the amount of help that an individual requires infers dependency?
3   It might be difficult to evaluate and compare the dependency levels of two patients, or even of the same patient at two different times. For example, unless further descriptive information was to be recorded, it would not be possible to ascertain whether the patient's level of *needing some help* has changed from what it had previously been.
4   The tool cannot be used to make comparative evaluations of levels/degrees of dependency or need. If *needing some help* scores 5 points and being *independent* scores 10 points, is someone who needs a little assistance with adjusting their clothing twice as dependent as someone who does not need such assistance? Is someone who is usually able to wipe themselves independently twice as dependent on the odd day when their arthritis is troubling them and they need some help?

A third example of an assessment tool is the Minimum Data Set (MDS) for nursing home residents in the USA.[13] This tool has many sections providing a wide spectrum of information about the nursing home patient. It uses questions of various constructions, but again most of them require the assessor to select the descriptor that most closely applies to their patient.

> **Box 2.5 Unsettled relationships[13]**
>
> *Check all that apply during the last seven days. If comatose, skip section.*
>
> - Covert/open conflict with and/or repeated criticism of staff
> - Unhappy with room mate
> - Unhappy with residents other than room mate
> - Openly expresses conflict/anger with family or friends
> - Absence of personal contact with family/friends
> - Recent loss of close family member/friend
> - None of above

Again, despite the potential benefits (*see* Table 2.1), there are also a number of potential problems with making judgements based on such criteria.[14]

1 The nurse may feel that none of the statements apply to their patient, but selects one anyway.
2 The nurse may feel that none of the statements apply to their patient, and leaves that section blank.
3 The nurse may feel that part of one statement and part of another statement provide the most accurate description of their patient. Do they select one or the other, both, or neither? Whichever option they choose, it is clear that the nurse's selection will not accurately describe the patient.
4 The nurse may not actually understand what the descriptors are saying or the point that they are making.

Some general concerns relating to the use of assessment tools

Concerns relating to specific assessment tool structures were outlined earlier. These are intended only to make the reader aware of issues relating to the use of assessment tools, and are certainly not intended as a direct criticism of individual tools. A more detailed critique of evaluating the use of a tool can be found on p. 14, but here are some more general concerns about the use of assessment tools.

1 Each nurse may interpret the statements in their own different way.
2 The nurse will need to involve the patient in the assessment if they are to be truly informed about the patient's status/behaviour/motivations (*see* Chapter 7 for ethical, professional and legal reasons why the nurse should always strive to do this). There are various reasons why this may not occur (*see* Chapter 6). This may therefore render the assessment outcome unreliable, and the process unethical, unprofessional and possibly illegal.
3 The nurse may have different perceptions of the patient's ability/needs to those of the patient him or herself.
4 When making the assessment the nurse will be relying on having the appropriate information to hand. If they have forgotten some observation that they have made of the patient (e.g. that he became rather aggressive earlier in the week), they will not include that observation in their assessment (*see* p. 52 for a detailed analysis of the role of the nurse's memory in assessment).

5 It is also possible that relevant patient information has not been communicated by other staff. No nurse is on duty 24 hours a day, seven days a week, and they will be reliant on information from other staff (*see* p. 63 for more information on how communication between nurses can influence the accuracy of assessment judgements). If they are not in possession of this information, they will be unable to make an informed judgement.

6 The nurse's judgement may be based on stereotypical, prejudiced or otherwise inaccurate perceptions of the patient (*see* Chapter 5).

Assessment tools and older adults

Much attention has been paid to the development of assessment tools specifically for use with older adults, in recognition of their often complex healthcare needs, and it is generally acknowledged that there are considerable advantages to using an assessment tool, rather than the nurse conducting their own informal or *ad hoc* assessment. However, there are also a number of disadvantages to the use of assessment tools in general, and I have already explored some of the issues relating to the use of specific types of tool. Table 2.1 provides a summary of the relative advantages and disadvantages of *ad hoc* (and also 'open') assessments and assessments conducted using a tool.

Making an assessment will rely on the nurse obtaining information about their patient (for a discussion of the processes of information acquisition, *see* Chapter 4). This information may be a direct result of the nurse's observations, or alternatively they may obtain information from patient notes or conversations with the patient, his or her relatives or other healthcare professionals (*see* Chapter 6). Assessments may be formal (e.g. when assessing for the level of Registered Nursing Care Contribution[20]), or they may be an informal response to an incident or change in the patient's condition.

Table 2.1 shows some of the advantages and disadvantages of both formal and informal assessments, and there is a lot for the nurse to consider. It would certainly appear that there are many disadvantages of using an assessment tool. Although there is a need to be aware of these, I would not want this to deter nurses from using them. Assessment tools, when used effectively, can positively enhance the consistent provision of patient-centred care, and may be used in conjunction with informal methods of assessment to provide an invaluable profile of the patient and their needs. Indeed, it has been acknowledged that both formal and informal assessments have their place – for example, in evaluating the risk of the patient developing pressure sores.[19]

Selecting a tool

An enormous amount of time and effort may go into developing and testing the reliability and validity of assessment tools, and they can have clear benefits for patient care. However, in my experience, such benefits will only be achieved if the following conditions are met.

1 The *appropriate* tool is selected.

2 The person responsible for selecting the tool has *researched it* carefully. They will need to consider both published and non-published evidence that the tool

Table 2.1 A comparison of the relative advantages and disadvantages of informal assessments of patient status/need and assessments using an assessment tool

	'Informal' assessment	*Assessment using an assessment tool*
Advantages	• The assessment can be completed quickly – on the spot – with no need for the nurse to collect specialised assessment documents • The assessment will be guided by and based on the nurse's own knowledge and experience • The nurse can tailor the assessment in response to perceived patient need • Nurses are not required to fit their evaluation of a patient into a pre-designed assessment format that may not be entirely suitable[15]	• The assessment tool may provide some useful guidelines or a framework for the conduct of the assessment[16] • May enable nurses to comply with clinical governance guidelines[16] • Using a specialist assessment tool may be useful for nurses less experienced in that particular area of care • It is possible that the use of an assessment tool will encourage nurses to document their patient evaluation • If a standardised assessment tool is used (e.g. the Waterlow Scale[17] for evaluating a patient's risk of developing pressure sores), this may permit comparison of the patient's current condition with that of other patients, or with previous/subsequent evaluations of the same patient made using the same scale
• Disadvantages	• The assessment may be highly subjective if guided by or based on the nurse's own knowledge and experience • An area of need may be 'forgotten' without the use of an assessment tool as a prompt • It would be difficult to compare the patient's current condition/healthcare status with prior/subsequent evaluations • It would be difficult to compare the patient's condition/healthcare status with that of other patients	• The assessment tool may be cumbersome and non-user friendly • The accuracy of the assessment may be impaired if nurses have not been trained to use the assessment tool[18] • Nurses may not understand some of the language and terminology used • The appropriate tool may not have been selected • The assessment format may be restrictive and actually limit the communication of pertinent patient information[15]

Table 2.1 (*cont.*)

'Informal' assessment	Assessment using an assessment tool
• The assessment will be based on the nurse's knowledge and expertise, and therefore possibly limited by any lack of knowledge or expertise • It would be very difficult to evaluate the reliability of the assessment • It would be very difficult to evaluate the validity of the assessment	• The validity of the tool may not have been tested. A tool is valid if it measures what it is meant to be measuring. For example, an oral thermometer is a valid means of measuring body temperature • The reliability of a tool may not have been tested. For a tool to be reliable it must consistently give the same result if used in the same conditions • The nurse may allow the tool to over-ride their own expert knowledge. For example, they may accept an assessment score indicating a very low risk of their patient developing a pressure sore, when in fact their own knowledge and experience might indicate the opposite. Indeed, the National Institute for Clinical Excellence[19] does acknowledge the sometimes poor predictive ability of pressure ulcer risk assessments,[21] and recommends that 'risk assessment tools should only be used as an aide-mémoire and should not replace clinical judgement' • Where assessment tools ask nurses to select from a number of statements describing their patient's condition/status, the nurse may find that none of the statements directly apply to their patient. There is evidence that nurses will still select a statement even if it does not accurately describe their patient[14]

is reliable and valid for use in their clinical area. Clear evidence will also be required that the tool has good inter-rater reliability – that is, different nurses using the same tool on the same patient at the same time will obtain similar assessment scores. Such investigations may take some time, but are advisable. As an illustrative example it is worth considering that Schoonhoven et al.[21] reviewed more than 40 scales for predicting the risk of patients developing pressure ulcers. Of these, only six had actually been tested for predictive validity. In other words, these scales had been devised on the basis of literature reviews or the opinions of experts, or adapted from other scales, but had *not been tested* to evaluate how valid their predictions were.

3 This investment is given the same *consideration* as any other financial investment. Assessment tools are usually purchased from the organisations that have developed them. A poor investment in this area will have both financial and human costs.
4 The nurses in the field are *committed* to using the tool.
5 The nurses in the field have been *trained* to use it.
6 The assessment is based on reliable and valid *information*, preferably with full *patient involvement* in the process.
7 The information obtained is actually used to *inform* the planning and delivery of care, and is not simply filed away neatly never to be looked at again.
8 The nurses use their *common sense* – if something does not seem right, check it out.

Older adults: a distinct client group?

This book focuses on the assessment of the healthcare needs of older adults, and by differentiating between this client group and others, it is implied that their needs differ. As the intended focus of this book is the regard of patients as individual human beings, it may therefore seem somewhat contradictory to view older adults as a homogenous concept. I very much want to avoid this wherever possible, but it has to be acknowledged that as a group, the needs of older adults differ from those of younger adults. Although many older adults live active and independent lives, free from illness, a significant proportion do need some form of healthcare intervention.[22] Indeed, 74% of women and 67% of men aged 85 years or older have some form of illness or disability that interferes with their ability to perform the activities of daily living. This compares with 26% of women and 27% of men aged between 50 and 64 years suffering the same degree of disability.[23]

It would therefore be unrealistic not to acknowledge that older adults are the main users of health and social care services,[24] and that normal ageing can be expected to be accompanied by degeneration, to varying degrees, of physical, physiological and psychological functioning. This may be accompanied by the effects of disease pathology, and exacerbated further by extraneous stressful life events such as the loss of a spouse.[22]

But what is an 'older adult'? Within healthcare, old age is determined not by how many years an individual has lived, but by the position that they assume on the continuum existing between the end of their working and child-rearing life and what is described as a state of frailty and dependency.[24] Indeed, Coupland

and Coupland[25] suggest that in Western societies there is a tendency to redefine ageing in terms of dependency on health and social services or a 'quasi-medical concern'[25] (p. 88). This is reflected in the way that the Department of Health classifies older people.[24] *The National Service Framework for Older People*[24] describes three stages of older age as 'entering old age', 'the transitional phase' and the 'frail older person'. Adults are said to have reached the initial phase of *entering old age* when they have:[24]

> Completed their career in paid employment and/or child rearing. This is a socially constructed definition of age which, according to different interpretations, includes people as young as 50, or from the official retirement ages of 60 for women and 65 for men. (p. 3)

This is a classification pertinent only in post-industrialised societies where significant numbers of individuals live beyond their working life,[26] and does bring with it the association of being beyond useful function.[25]

Defining old age is difficult, and as already stated it may be interpreted on the basis of a factor such as an individual's occupation. Furthermore, a person's attitudes and appearance may induce others to consider them 'old',[22] while the number of years since they were born might indicate otherwise. I am sure that all readers are familiar with statements such as 'I thought that she was older than that – she certainly looks it!' or 'He's had his hair cut – it's taken years off him', where inferences are made about people's ages on the basis of how they look.

Therefore, although the diverse nature of older adulthood has been asserted, the special needs of some members of this group cannot be denied.[24] As these needs are commonly allied to age-related physiological, sociological and psychological changes,[22] consideration of the nursing needs of older adults as a group is the most practical and feasible option for the purpose of this book. In other words, although I am keen not to project a stereotypical image of all older people as being dependent, in ill health and generally frail, I would be unrealistic if I did not acknowledge that a proportion of them are.

Why might assessment of an older adult be difficult?

Assessment of the older adult is fraught with difficulty.[27] Complex health problems may arise, associated with age-related mortality and pathologies.[24] For example, establishing validity and reliability can be difficult in people with depression or cognitive impairment.[27] The assessment may rely even more heavily on the subjective input of assessors who may lack the necessary skills and awareness.[18] They may be unaware of how cognitive and perceptual degeneration may influence the reliability of the assessment, or how the complex interaction of age- and non-age-related factors might affect the health status of an individual. Nurses may lack the necessary skills and knowledge to recognise health needs in their early stages, and many older people may receive inappropriate care due to inadequate assessment of their abilities and needs.[28]

The person being assessed may be unable[27] or unwilling[18] to contribute to the assessment process. The patient may dislike or distrust the nurse and be influenced by their communication skills (or lack of them) or by their conduct. Those making an assessment of an older adult will need to have the awareness, insight and knowledge to make an accurate and informed assessment.[4,29] They need to be sensitive to any indicators that all is not well with the patient. For example, they might notice that the patient has small burns on their hands from cooking, or bruising from a fall. Odours may indicate that the patient is experiencing urinary incontinence, or the patient's clothes may appear a little too large, indicating that they have lost weight. If these cues are missed at contact assessment, and the individual does not ask for help, then their needs may remain unrecognised.

The difficulty of obtaining a comprehensive assessment of nursing home residents is not disputed.[30] Much recent research interest has been focused on the establishment of a specific assessment tool's reliability and validity.[30,31] A reliable and valid assessment tool can provide a useful framework both for the organisation of data collection, and for the interpretation of information gathered. The developers of the Minimum Data Set (MDS),[13] a nationally implemented assessment tool for nursing homes in the USA, cite one of the aims of its introduction as being that 'the MDS should replace non-uniform and cursory assessment' (p. 294). However, Valk et al.[30] advise that attempting to achieve comprehensiveness in assessment by combining a number of instruments might make the assessment long, unwieldy and suitable only for use by skilled practitioners.

It should be appreciated that, regardless of the quality of the tool used, the accuracy of the assessment outcome will be determined by the quality of the information upon which it is based. Hawes et al.[27] indicate that measurement of the functional status of older adults, specifically those resident in nursing homes, presents specific challenges which include cognitive impairment and problems with communication. Not only may there be problems with the communication of information, but these patients' status and ability to communicate their needs may also vary over the assessment period,[27,30] or in response to those making the assessment.

Davies et al.[32] conducted a review of the relevant literature and concluded that if patients are to be afforded a maximum level of independence and autonomy, then their nursing care must accommodate their own particular and individual needs. Effective assessment and subsequent individualised care planning are a necessary component of this.[29] Potential inhibitors of an accurate assessment will be explored in greater detail in Chapters 2, 5 and 6.

The political context: assessment reforms

There have been significant reforms in the funding and assessment of care needs of the older adult. These have largely been initiated by the publication of *The NHS Plan*,[33] and heralded by the publication of the *National Service Framework for Older People* (NSFOP) in 2001[24] (for further information relating to this, *see* p. 23).

The NSFOP acknowledges that many older people have complex health and social care needs, and highlights the concern that there has been a lack of consistency in the assessment of older people. An individual who requires care of some kind may undergo one or more separate assessments by each member of the care team whom they encounter. These may include doctors, nurses, health visitors, physiotherapists, social workers, occupational therapists and continence advisers. Some information may be given repeatedly, while other information (and therefore possible needs) may be totally neglected. There may also be ineffective communication between care professionals.

The Single Assessment Process (SAP)[34] applies to health and social services, and was introduced from April 2002 (to be implemented by authorities by April 2004[35]) in response to the recommendations of the NSFOP. The aims of the SAP are to increase patient involvement in the planning of their care and to eliminate the need for repetition of assessments and information giving. The assessment of an individual's care needs, and planning for the provision of this care, will be achieved by means of a four-level assessment process. Instead of separate assessments, one amalgamated assessment is now completed and added to by individual health and social care providers, preferably in partnership with the patient.[24]

The need for quality assurance and consistency in the provision of care and the need to 'cost' the registered nursing care of older adults as part of the 'Free Nursing Care' initiative[20] were other reasons cited for effective assessment of the older adult.

In summary

A review of the literature indicates the difficulties and potential dangers encountered when defining and classifying older adults as a group. However, care needs specific to this group have been identified. The acknowledgement of this has resulted in the government focusing attention on the importance of effective assessment of the care needs of older adults. The concept of assessment has been explored, and despite the concerns relating to assessment raised in Chapter 1 and in this chapter, the general consensus is that if patients are to receive quality and individualised care, there first has to be an effective assessment of their needs.[4,18,29,32,36] Potential difficulties with regard to achieving an effective assessment have been outlined, and will be investigated in greater detail later in this book.

Key points

- Assessment should be an ongoing process, rather than a 'one-off' event, and it should be responsive to changes in a patient's needs or status.
- Employing an assessment tool will only benefit patient care if the appropriate tool is selected and staff are trained to use it.
- It should not be assumed that all older adults will be frail and dependent on input from healthcare services, but nurses should be aware of the special needs of some members of this group.
- Assessment of older adults may be difficult, and nurses need to be aware of and sympathetic to the special needs of this client group.

References

1 Royal College of Nursing (1997) *Royal College of Nursing Assessment Tool For Nursing Older People.* Royal College of Nursing, London.
2 Aggleton P and Chalmers H (2000) *Nursing Models and Nursing Practice* (2e). Macmillan, Basingstoke.
3 Roper N, Logan W and Tierney A (1983) *Using a Model for Nursing.* Churchill Livingstone, Edinburgh.
4 Heath H (2000) Assessing older people. *Elderly Care.* **11:** 27–8.
5 Philp I and Dunleavy J (1994) Community health assessment of elderly people: the national picture. *Health Soc Care Commun.* **12:** 117–19.
6 Philp I (1997) Can a medical and social assessment be combined? *J R Soc Med.* **90 (Suppl. 32):** 11–13.
7 Leuckenotte AG (1998) *Gerontologic Assessment* (3e). Mosby, St. Louis, MO.
8 Department of Health (2002) *The Single Assessment Process: assessment tools and scales;* www.doh.gov.uk/scg/sap/toolsandscales (accessed 12/12/02).
9 Folstein M, Folstein S and McHugh PR (1975) Mini-Mental State: a practical method for grading the cognitive state of patients for the clinician. *J Psychiatr Res.* **12:** 189–98.
10 Mahoney FI and Barthel D (1965) Functional evaluation: the Barthel Index. *Md Med J.* **14:** 56–61.
11 *The Barthel Index;* www.Strokecenter.org.trials/Scales/barthel.pdf (accessed 23/02/03).
12 Bowling A (2001) *Measuring Disease.* Open University Press, Buckingham.
13 Morris JN *et al.* (1990) Designing the National Resident Assessment Instrument for nursing homes. *Gerontologist.* **30:** 293–307.
14 Taylor H (2005) *The nursing assessment of older adults.* PhD thesis (unpublished), University College Worcester.
15 Baldwin S and Woods PA (1994) Case management and needs assessment: some issues of concern for the caring professions. *J Ment Health.* **3:** 311–22.
16 Franks PJ, Moffatt CJ and Chaloner D (2003) Risk assessment scales poorly predict pressure ulceration. *BMJ.* **326:** 165.
17 Waterlow J (1985) Pressure sores: a risk assessment card. *Nurs Times.* **81:** 49–55.
18 Richardson J (2001) The easy-care assessment system and its appropriateness for older people. *Nursing Older People.* **13:** 17–19.
19 National Institute for Clinical Excellence (2001) *Pressure Ulcer Risk Assessment and Prevention. Inherited clinical guideline B.* National Institute for Clinical Excellence, London.
20 Department of Health (2001) *NHS-Funded Nursing Care. Practice guide and workbook.* Department of Health, London.
21 Schoonhoven L *et al.* (2002) Prospective cohort study of routine use of risk assessment scales for prediction of pressure ulcers. *BMJ.* **325:** 797–801.
22 Stuart-Hamilton I (2000) *The Psychology of Ageing: an introduction* (3e). Jessica Kingsley Publishers, London.
23 National Statistics (2004) *Older People: health and caring;* www.statistics.gov.uk/cci/nscl.asp
24 Department of Health (2001) *National Service Framework for Older People.* Department of Health, London.
25 Coupland N and Coupland J (1995) Discourse, identity, and aging. In: JF Nussbaum and J Coupland (eds) *The Handbook of Communication and Aging Research.* Lawrence Erlbaum Associates, Inc., Mahwah, NJ.
26 Bromley DB (1988) *Human Ageing* (3e). Penguin, Harmondsworth.
27 Hawes C *et al.* (1995) Reliability estimates for the minimum data set for nursing home resident assessment and care screening (MDS). *Gerontologist.* **35:** 172–8.
28 Ford P (2001) A fair deal for older people. *Prim Health Care.* **11:** 37–41.

29 Challis D *et al.* (2004) The value of specialist clinical assessment of older people prior to entry to care homes. *Age Ageing*, **33:** 25–34.

30 Valk M *et al.* (2001) Measuring disability in nursing home residents: validity and reliability of a newly developed instrument. *J Gerontol B Psychol Sci Soc Sci.* **56:** 187–91.

31 Keller HH, McKenzie JD and Goy RE (2001) Construct validation and test–retest reliability of the seniors in the community: risk evaluation for eating and nutrition questionnaire. *J Gerontol Med Sci.* **56A:** M552–8.

32 Davies S, Laker S and Ellis L (1997) Promoting autonomy and independence for older people within nursing practice: a literature review. *J Adv Nurs.* **26:** 408–17.

33 Department of Health (2000) *The NHS Plan: a plan for investment, a plan for reform.* The Stationery Office, London.

34 Department of Health (2001) *The Single Assessment Process: consultation papers and process.* Department of Health, London.

35 www.dh.gov.uk/PolicyAndGuidance/HealthAndSocialCareTopics/SocialCare/Single AssessmentProcess/fs/en

36 Taylor H (2004) *The nursing assessment of older adults.* Conference proceedings of the Royal College of Nursing International Nursing Research Conference, 24 March, University of Cambridge, Cambridge.

Chapter 3

Defining 'registered nursing care' and 'nursing needs'

Background

Recent central and local government publications[1–4] have, in addition to reforms in the assessment and funding of those older adults receiving or entering long-term care, focused attention on the specific role of the registered nurse. The Health and Social Care Act[2] specifies that 'registered nursing care' should be free at the point of delivery for all those in receipt of continuing care, regardless of the setting within which they receive that care. In the past, those individuals who were funding their own care in nursing homes were charged for the input of a registered nurse. However, from 1 October 2001 these people were entitled to an allowance commensurate with their assessed need for registered nursing care. In order for this to be achieved, there must first be an assessment of an individual's registered nursing needs. Primary care trusts (PCTs) are now responsible for the appointment and training of nurses to assess and band patients according to the level of their registered nursing care needs – that is, to establish the Registered Nursing Care Contribution (RNCC).[5]

However, in the years since the implementation of the 'Free Nursing Care' initiative, a number of flaws have come to light. These relate mainly to a lack of uniformity in national assessment systems, and therefore inconsistency in the evaluation of patient need. This means that a patient may be judged by one authority to be in a 'high' band of need, yet a patient in a neighbouring authority with commensurate needs may be assessed and placed in a lower dependency band.[6]

In addition, although the Department of Health[5] describes specific domains for assessment of nursing need identified within the Single Assessment Process (SAP) (e.g. the senses, mental health, personal care and physical well-being), it makes no detailed prescription of assessment criteria for calculating the Registered Nursing Care Contribution. This establishes how much care an individual requires from a registered nurse, rather than from unqualified caregivers such as healthcare assistants. This means that difficulties may arise for those being cared for in a care home, defined by the Department of Health[7] as 'an establishment providing accommodation with nursing or personal care' (p. 45). Residents of care homes may receive care from both registered nurses and unqualified care assistants. Care from a registered nurse will be funded and provided either directly by the nurse, or by an unqualified care assistant under the nurse's supervision.

But how is 'nursing care' defined? The glossary of the *Care Homes for Older People: national minimum standards*[7] lists definitions of terms such as 'assisted bath' and 'procedure', but does not include 'nurse' or 'nursing care'. 'Personal care' was defined as 'care which includes assistance with bodily functions when required' (p. 46), yet this does not differentiate between assistance given by nurses, care assistants and informal carers.[8] Thus although the Department of Health has advocated the importance of delivering quality 'nursing care',[5] there is no definition of exactly what this constitutes. However, the Department does provide some clarification of what registered nursing care is not:[5]

> This [registered nursing care] does not include time spent by non-nursing staff such as care assistants (although it does cover the nurse time spent in monitoring or supervising care that is delegated to others), neither does it cover personal or social care costs or the costs of accommodation to residents. (p. 3)

The Royal Commission on Long-Term Care[9] has added to the confusion somewhat by suggesting that nursing care 'involves the knowledge or skills of a qualified nurse', without specifying what the knowledge and skills might be. They also make a distinction between 'nursing' and 'personal care', yet the definition of the latter as care that 'falls within the internationally recognised definition of nursing, but may be delivered by many people who are not nurses, in particular by care assistants' (paragraph 6.43) does little to make the difference explicit.[8] Neither the Nursing and Midwifery Council[10] nor the Department of Health[5] has provided definitive criteria for registered nursing care. This may be because of a perception of the nurse role as being flexible, metamorphic and responsive to individual environmental and professional demands:[10]

> 6.2 – To practise competently, you must possess the knowledge, skills and abilities required for lawful, safe and effective practice without direct supervision . . .
> 6.3 – If an aspect of practice is beyond your level of competence or outside your area of registration, you must obtain help and supervision from a competent practitioner until you and your employer consider that you have acquired the requisite knowledge and skill. (p. 9)

It is likely that as nurses have assumed more of the roles that were traditionally undertaken by doctors – that is, prescribing, making direct referrals, running clinics, minor surgery, and so on – duties once performed by registered nurses have been assumed by others, including healthcare assistants and informal carers.[8,11] Changes in the nurse's role, with the introduction of initiatives such as the expanded role, nurse practitioners and nurse consultants,[12] may therefore make it unhelpful to conclude that 'nursing is what nurses do',[8] without being able to answer questions such as 'which nurses?' and 'where?'. It would be reasonable to assume that 'what nurses do' depends very much on where they are working, their level of expertise and the demands that are placed on them.

The work of registered nurses is also regarded as being more than care that they physically deliver themselves, and can in addition involve the supervision and management of unqualified staff.[13] It may therefore be asked 'To what extent does a nurse have to contribute to an act for it to become a nursing task, and at what point does a task traditionally performed by others (e.g. doctors) become a nursing task if adopted by nurses?'.[8] Indeed, the Health Service Ombudsman reiterated the difficulties in defining 'nursing care',[6] suggesting that:

> The distinction between health and social care (and that care by registered nurses or by others) is a blurred one which has also shifted over time. Nurses have been trained to take on tasks which years ago would only have been carried out by doctors, and auxiliary nurses, care assistants and carers increasingly perform tasks which, in the past, would have been carried out only by registered nurses.   (p. 7)

But why is the ability to define registered nursing so important? First let us consider this question from a professional perspective. It has been suggested that in order for nursing to establish itself as a discrete profession, practising nurses need to be able to:[14]

> accurately define, with a high degree of specification, those particular areas of concern in healthcare clients for which they, as nurses, are uniquely qualified to offer solutions.   (p. 185)

In other words, nurses need to be able to clearly state exactly what services, skills or knowledge registered nurses, and *only* registered nurses, can provide. A number of broad issues have been suggested, including specialist knowledge informing an assessment of patient need, clinical judgement, personal account-ability for their actions (including those delegated to others), and the ethically and professionally regulated relationship between nurse and patient.[8,11] How-ever, there is no professional or legal scope for any nurse to be able to state that they and only they may perform a given care function.

A need for such definition is also significant from a patient care perspective. Although it has been stated in the previous paragraph that an ability specific to nurses was 'specialist knowledge informing an assessment of patient need', how is it possible to assess for nursing care needs without first knowing what the boundaries of registered nursing are? It is likely that both individual nurses and groups of nurses have clear ideas about their role, but how useful is this when considering wider issues such as the government initiatives relating to assessment and care of older adults? Each group of nurses or each individual nurse could feasibly have their own way of approaching assessment. As an illustrative example, consider the potential differences in practice for a team of community nurses working in a rural Welsh district, and a group of staff nurses working on a medical assessment unit in an inner-city area. Although there will be many similarities, there are also likely to be some differences in the daily challenges faced by these two nurse groups, and these may influence their approaches to nursing care and thus assessment of patient need. These will be dependent on how the nurses perceive their own role and other factors that will be explored in the remainder of this chapter.

It is also likely that there will be some lack of insight and understanding both intra- and interprofessionally with regard to the work that each nurse group undertakes, with the work of a nurse in a nursing home possibly differing from that of a nurse in a secondary care setting. Indeed, it has been shown that acute hospital nurses may have limited understanding of the work done within the aged care system.[15] So what are nursing tasks? There is scope for disparity in the perception of the nurse's role, and if nurses are unable to define what nurses 'do', then the potential difficulties in assessing registered nursing need are clear.

The patient's perspective

It is also possible that there will be differences in the perceptions of nurses and their patients about what constitutes the nurse's role, and this may result in differences in expectations of the care that nurses deliver. Research studies have supported this and are explored in more detail in Chapter 6. Some examples include differences in what patients and nurses regard as important, with research by Milne and McWilliam[16] indicating that whereas patients valued the nurse simply spending time with them and being with them, nurses tended to spend time 'just being' with the patient only when other, and what they considered to be more essential, nursing work had been completed. This suggests a discrepancy in nurse and patient values, and differences in what patients and nurses expect of a nursing service.

It has also been indicated that there is conflict between nurses' perceptions of what is important for their older patients, and what the patients themselves consider to be important.[17] In addition, there is a suggestion that a patient's sense of what is important to them may vary with their level of dependency.[18] There are also differences between different patient groups, with research indicating that older adults are generally more satisfied with NHS services than younger people.[1] One possible explanation for this could be that these people remember the inadequacies of healthcare services that existed before the introduction of the NHS and the modern welfare state. They may therefore generally have lower expectations than younger people and demand less from nurses (*see* Chapter 6).

Self-concept and nurse role

Brykczynska,[19] in her exploration of the meaning of the term 'nursing values', expounds the importance of 'values' to those working within the healthcare professions, 'because it is precisely how we think and feel about issues and aspects of life that ultimately governs our behaviour' (p. 131). But what are values? The *Concise Oxford English Dictionary* describes 'values' as being 'principles or standards of behaviour'. Within a professional context, Banks[20] suggests that values refer to the 'fundamental moral/ethical principles' (p. 6) to which members of that profession are committed. Although her comments are specifically allied to the work of social workers, it is useful to relate this to nursing practice and to suggest that the latter may be shaped and influenced both by a nurse's own values and by societal and professional values. Banks[20] argues that the 'good' social worker (the reflective practitioner[21]) needs to be 'aware of the societal and professional values underlying her work and her own values, and should adopt a critical stance to her practice' (p. 64). She relates this to assessment. For example, factual knowledge of what assessment is, or what needs are, will be shaped and influenced by an individual's values. However, she continues by asserting that:

> This is not to say that in order for a social worker to be able to do an
> assessment of a user's needs she has to know what concept of need the
> assessment is based upon, just that any assessment of need pre-

supposes some concept of what need is, and this will be an evaluative concept. The doing of the assessment is not 'value-neutral', even if the social worker is simply filling in a form designed by someone else.

(p. 64)

It may be inferred from this that a nurse's values, societal values and professional values will all have an impact on the assessment process.

Ajzen and Fishbein[22] have explored what are collectively known as 'consistency theories'. They have evaluated the relationship between how an individual behaves, and their beliefs and attitudes towards that behaviour. The consensus appears to be that individuals strive to achieve consistency between their beliefs, attitudes and behaviours.[22] However, although their review of the research findings in this area indicates that people tend to bring their beliefs and attitudes into line with their actions, they provide no information about the extent to which attitudes influence behaviour.[22] People tend to behave in a manner that is consistent with their beliefs and attitudes, but the extent to which behaviour is thus influenced remains unclear.[22]

Arthur[23] postulates that 'the "professional" self-concept of nurses is unique and different from that of the self-concept (whilst inextricably linked)' (p. 712). He argues that nurses need a professional self-identity that is compatible with other healthcare professionals with whom they work. He suggests that if nurses have a low self-concept, then senior nurse managers and nurse academics should address this, and he proposes that elevation of status and regard for nurses would result in an improved professional self-concept. He considers that such a positive self-identity is essential if nurses are to assume:[23]

> more responsibility and accountability for nursing care. While it could be argued that a well-developed professional self-concept will assist the delivery of this care, as well as improving the individual nurse's personal self-concept, including self-confidence and self-respect.

(p. 712)

Arthur[23] assumes that self-identity and professional identity, although linked, are separate entities, and also that there will be a correlation between a nurse's perception of the 'ideal professional' and their own professional self-concept. He adopts Burns' definition of self-concept[24] as a 'relatively enduring organisation of affective and evaluative beliefs about oneself predisposing one to respond with greater probability in one way than in another' (p. 713). Furthermore, he suggests that in order for individuals to regard and accept themselves positively, they must have a positive self-concept, as a negative self-concept would evoke a converse, negative perception of self.

A major concern is the use of terms such as 'self-concept' and 'self-esteem', with Strein[25] in his review of the literature identifying in excess of 15 'self-terms', often used interchangeably, and often relating to different ways in which people view themselves. Of particular relevance are the terms 'self-concept', 'self-worth', 'self-esteem' and 'self-acceptance'. Elliott[26] argues that Rosenberg has made one of the most significant contributions to self-concept and self-esteem theory. Rosenberg[27] describes 'self-concept' as 'the totality of the individual's thoughts and feelings having reference to himself as an object' (p. 7). Furthermore, Goodman's review[28] of Rosenberg's work identifies that the drive for positive self-esteem is a significant motivator of an individual's actions and behaviour, and thus distinct from self-concept, defined as a perception of or attitude towards oneself.

Ervin and Stryker[29] make a postulation, based on Rosenberg's theory, that 'people are selective in which roles, which aspects of a role, and which qualities relevant to a role they emphasise' (p. 48) in order to present a positive image of themselves. An individual will have their own idea of what aspects of their world are important to them and how they view themselves. The degree of importance that they ascribe to a particular role will depend on what is significant in order to either maintain or promote a positive self-concept. On the basis of this, Arthur's distinction of professional and self-concepts as two separate entities does appear inappropriate.

When consistency theories and the theory of the relationship between self-concept, self-esteem and behaviour are considered together, it could be said that if a nurse is to promote positive self-esteem and thus self-concept, they would be motivated to adopt a professional role that fulfils their expectations of the importance of a particular role. This may influence their perception of what a nurse is and does, and thus their assessment of a patient's need for nursing care. For example, if helping a patient to get washed and dressed promotes negative self-concept in a nurse, then if they are in a position to choose, it is possible that they would disregard this as part of their professional role. When assessing a patient's specific nursing needs, their ability to wash and dress may thus be disregarded, as the nurse does not consider this area of care to be part of their professional role.

In pursuit of higher status?

Phillips[30] explores a 'tension between the generally accepted theoretical move towards holism in healthcare and the practical reality of applying holistic healthcare in a society which continues to hold the scientific/biomedical paradigm in high regard' (p. 139). She expounds concern 'about the wider social and political implications of emotional labour in healthcare, with particular reference to women and their position in society'. She exposes the conflict experienced by a profession which, while valuing the emotional/caring component of care, faces the reality of trying to elevate its status in a 'modern scientific society' (p. 142). In other words, although nurses recognise the importance of the 'caring' aspects of their work, they may also perceive that society does not hold this in such high regard as the more technical aspects of their work.

It could be argued that changes in nursing practice, such as the assumption of more technical tasks and the delegation of what some may regard as more menial tasks (e.g. helping patients to fulfil their personal hygiene needs) to healthcare assistants, resulted from a desire to improve professional self-concept. Indeed, Barnard and Sandelowski[31] postulate that although nurses have sought to establish professional identity by distancing themselves from medicine and 'technology', at the same time they have accepted technical tasks delegated to them in an attempt to elevate their professional status. These authors go on to suggest that for a professional group that has 'never established fully a separate and secure identity, it is the abandonment of divisions – not the divisions themselves – that may seem precarious and arbitrary' (p. 373).

Barnard and Sandelowski[31] contest the assumption implicit in this that there is a boundary between 'caring' and the performance of technical tasks. Indeed, they argue that:

> What determines whether a technology dehumanises, depersonalises or objectifies is not technology *per se*, but rather how individual technologies operate in specific user contexts, the meanings attributed to them, how any one individual or cultural group defines what is human. . . . Humane care is itself a socially constructed entity.
>
> (p. 372)

On the basis of this, if nurses have worked to establish professional identity by distancing themselves from medicine – by establishing and asserting the differences between the medical and caring models – then this should be considered to be an artificial distinction. This has been based on the unfounded assumption that 'technical' tasks or those more traditionally associated with the medical profession are conducted in the absence of caring.[31]

Barnard and Sandelowski[31] put the assertions of Ellul[32] into context. They suggest that within professional discourse there is often too much emphasis on differences that do not exist or that are irrelevant:[31] 'More talk of freedom often means there is less freedom, more talk of respect, less respect, and more talk of humane care, less humane care' (p. 373). Such a focus, they suggest, would detract from differences or issues that really do matter. Such emphasis may further confuse definitions of nursing and the nursing role.

What are nursing needs?

The discussion concerning the definition of the nursing role is central to the main concern of this book, namely nursing assessment. It could be argued that a nurse would only assess for nursing needs based on their own consideration of what constitutes their role as a nurse. It has been established that role determination will be influenced by a number of factors (e.g. a desire to achieve positive self-esteem), so there will be some flexibility in how individual nurses determine their nursing role. Therefore if a nurse considers that an element of care does not constitute 'nursing care', it could be said that they would not recognise this as a nursing need. For a nurse to assess for nursing need, it must first be recognised as fitting the remit of nursing care. This is supported by Jones' definition of 'nursing diagnosis' as being the recognition and identification of cues given by a patient indicating that they have a need for nursing input.[14] For a nurse to recognise and assess a patient's need for nursing care, the nurse must first acknowledge that this need falls within what they consider to be the realm of nursing.

It has already been established that the role of a nursing assessment is to identify nursing needs (*see* Chapter 2), and thus to provide a basis for individualised nursing care.[13] But what is a 'need'? There is a variety of nursing models, each differing in some manner in the assumptions that it makes about the health-related needs of individuals.[33] The word 'need' is used frequently throughout this book, usually within the context of 'nursing need'. But what does it mean? Liss[34] suggests that the word 'need' implies some form of suffering, and that caring for a person will be in response to that person's needs. He defines an individual as having a healthcare need 'in so far as his or her actual state of health is considered unsatisfactory with regard to the optimal state of health' (p. 17). However, this definition fails to define who determines the need and upon which criteria.

Sheaff[35] asserts that 'we pursue our needs for healthcare through the cycle of drive, action and satisfaction' (p. 106), and that as individuals we are usually able to do this without considerable help from healthcare professionals. When healthcare problems arise, then so may healthcare needs. However, what the patient does not require are healthcare professionals to perform tasks that they are able to perform for themselves (*see* Chapter 6 for further information on imposed and learned dependency in patients[36]). Sheaff goes on to argue that the 'mentally healthy patient', aided by the specialist knowledge of the doctor or other healthcare professional, will be best able to determine these needs.

The use of the word 'need' implies that an individual has some kind of deficit which may be remedied in some way.[35] This need may be for knowledge, for physical intervention by another or for the physical replacement of some missing factor. Lockward and Marshall[37] suggest that the 'needs-led' approach to care was a reaction against what they consider to be the 'medical approach' whereby care needs were defined by an individual's medical diagnosis. They cite nurse theorists such as Peplau,[38] who believed that such an approach fails to adequately address an individual's holistic care needs. Lockward and Marshall[37] propose that such a reaction to the 'medical approach', and a move towards what they regard as a holistic assessment of needs, has been influential in the development of both nursing and social models of care.

Nursing models usually specify how the nurse, working in collaboration with the patient, may work to assess and thereby identify these needs. For example, Neuman[39] advocated identifying areas where stressors (internal and external) threaten or have actually penetrated the individual's 'lines of defence'. By working with the individual, the nurse may help them to prevent, restore or maintain their adaptation to these stressors, and unnecessary care is not inflicted on the individual. The patient and nurse work together to identify both the patient's needs and how they may be addressed.[37]

Because the terms 'need' and 'nursing need' are used throughout this book, there is some requirement for their meaning to be established. The terms 'nursing need' or 'care need' are taken to mean that an individual has some form of deficit identified either by him- or herself or by a third party which requires intervention from a nurse or other healthcare provider in partnership and in collaboration with him or her. The aim of this intervention will be to minimise the impact of any actual or potential health deficits.

How do individual nurses interpret the nurse's role?

A study by Chang and Twinn[40] indicates that nurses may vary in their perception of the nurse's role, both with regard to level of seniority and in relation to their work location.[41] However, many decisions about nursing and health policy are made by individuals who are not nurses, or by nurses without expertise in that particular field. For example, the Secretary of State for Health at the time this book was written, Dr John Reid, has an educational background in history and has held office in the Ministries of Transport and Defence.[42] It could reasonably be said that his expertise in diverse fields might influence the way in which he regards health and the provision of healthcare. Those outside the discipline (e.g. family and friends) may influence the nurse's perception of what is appropriate.

Care for an older adult is delivered in a variety of quite different settings[43] (e.g. privately run nursing homes and NHS hospitals), and there is a possibility that perceptions of the nurse's role may also relate to the institution in which they work. It is not clear, for example, whether there are differences with regard to what tasks are considered appropriate for a registered nurse providing care for older adults in a nursing home and on an NHS medical ward. If there is a difference, this may have implications for the definition of role for registered nurses working in these loci, and therefore their evaluation of what constitutes an individual's nursing needs. Should this be true, it is also possible that there would be differences in nurse assessment practice between work loci.

The implications of this are important, because although the need for effective assessment of the nursing needs of older adults has been asserted, there remains no consensus of opinion as to what 'nursing care' is. The determination of needs would not be value free, and will be vulnerable to the individual perceptions of all those involved in the care process (*see* Chapters 3 and 6), such as the government, the nursing profession, patients and individual nurses. For nurses, this may be shaped by factors such as their own experiences, education and a desire to achieve positive self-esteem in their professional role. For a nurse to assess a nursing need, they must first accept that such a need would fall within what they consider to be the nursing domain.[14]

I conducted an investigation into perceptions of the nurse's role, specifically to explore the perceived 'appropriateness' of a registered nurse performing 28 defined tasks while providing care for older adults.[8,44] The study had three objectives:

1 to investigate whether there are role expectations linked to the nurse's work locus
2 to compare what both nurses and non-nurses consider to be appropriate tasks for a registered nurse to perform
3 to gain some insight into how the nurse's role is perceived.

A self-administered questionnaire survey asked a sample of 145 undergraduates in healthcare and non-healthcare subjects, teachers and practising nurses to comment on the appropriateness of a number of tasks performed by a nurse called Sarah during the course of an eight-hour shift that involved caring for older adults. The respondents received one of two versions of the questionnaire. In one version Sarah worked in a nursing home, and in the other she worked on a hospital ward. Respondents were also asked to comment on a number of statements relating to nursing in general. The findings suggest that as a consequence of assuming 'technical tasks', there has been some elevation of status for the nursing profession, yet the importance of 'hands-on' nursing tasks remains valid. This would suggest that nursing and the work that individual nurses do are seen to involve a complex interplay of tasks.[44] The findings also indicate that there are differences in the perceived roles of nurses providing care for older adults in nursing homes and in NHS hospitals.

Although this was a small-scale study, with a number of methodological limitations (e.g. a small proportion of nurse respondents compared with lay respondents), it does raise some interesting points concerning perceptions of the nurse's role and assessment.

1   The tasks that respondents considered appropriate for the registered nurse to perform were dependent upon work locus. These perceptions were also related to the source of the respondent's information about nurses and the work that they do. There were some differences between the responses of nurses and non-nurses. It may therefore be concluded that the role of the registered nurse working in a nursing home is perceived to be different from that of the registered nurse working with the same client group on a general hospital ward. If nurses do indeed expect the nursing work in a nursing home to differ from that in a hospital, it is conceivable that nurse assessment of patient needs in these two areas will differ.
2   A non-nursing individual's perceptions of nurses and the work that they do is often influenced by the way in which nurses are portrayed in the media, and by their observations of nurses working with other people. Patients and their relatives may therefore have expectations of nursing care that are not grounded in reality. Expectations of patients and their relatives may influence their contribution to the assessment process.
3   Although it was agreed that 'hands-on care' represented good use of nursing skills, it was also asserted that the acquisition of 'technical tasks' and the delegation of 'more routine patient care tasks' have improved the status of nursing. If nurses are motivated to achieve positive self-esteem, how far do they actively seek to adopt a nursing role that is sympathetic to this? And will there be a difference in the assessment of nursing needs between nurses working in nursing homes and those working in hospitals?

These findings provide an important insight into our understanding of the nurse's role. The perceptions of nurses and others around them will contribute significantly to the way in which an individual nurse conceptualises their role. This view is supported by the theory of 'reasoned action', in which a nurse's personal attitudes and their 'subjective norm'[22] influence their intent to perform that behaviour (*see* Figure 3.1). Given that Ajzen and Fishbein[22] define subjective norm as 'a person's belief that most of her important others think she should (or should not) perform the behaviour in question' (p. 73), the nurse may have been influenced by their nurse educators,[45] their nursing and non-nursing colleagues, their patients, their families and the media. According to this model, these may all

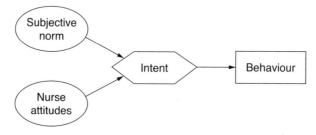

Figure 3.1 Intention to perform behaviour.[23]

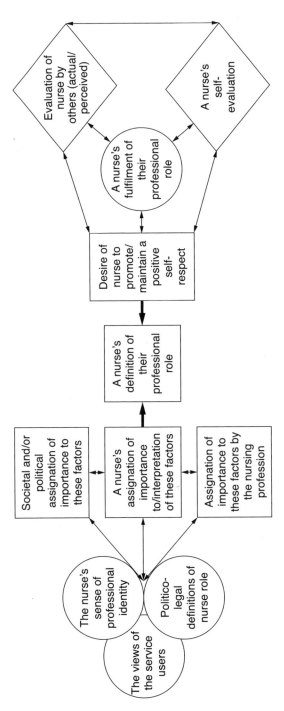

Figure 3.2 Factors that affect an individual nurse's definition of professional role.

impact on how individual nurses conceptualise their nursing role, and therefore determine their nursing behaviour.

Consider the model outlined in Figure 3.2. I devised this on the basis of both research findings[44] and the literature reviewed earlier in this chapter, and it relates the factors that may influence an individual nurse's definition of their professional role. This role definition may be based on a complex interplay of a number of factors, including the nurse's sense of professional identity (the definitions and a construct imposed by the nursing profession on how the nursing role is defined), the views of the service users (the general public – both individuals and groups), and politico-legal definitions of the nurse's role. As indicated by research findings,[44] these will all be open to interpretation by society in general, by the nursing profession and by nurses themselves. The nurse will also be receptive to how they interpret and value the views of the groups mentioned. In addition to the nurse's own values,[19] these in turn will influence and shape the nurse's definition of their role, and thus motivate their desire to promote and/or maintain a positive self-concept.

The nurse's fulfilment of their professional role will be subject to self-evaluation and the actual or perceived evaluation of others (e.g. peers, service users or nurse managers). An individual nurse's definition of their role will therefore be distinct from that of any other nurse. If nurses all have different perceptions of role, or intent to perform behaviours specific to their nursing role, it could be said that a nurse's assessments of patient need would be shaped by his or her perception of the nurse's role within a care domain (*see* Figure 3.3). For example, if a nurse considers it inappropriate for a registered nurse to assist a patient in selecting their clothes, it is possible that they would not consider it necessary to assess that patient's ability to select their own clothes.

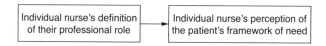

Figure 3.3 The influence of role on perceptions of need.

They may disregard an area of care that they regard as either unimportant or irrelevant. The nurse will confine their assessment to areas of care within what they consider to be the nursing domain, whether it is the direct provision of care or care provided by others under the supervision of the nurse.

Taking together consistency theories and the theory of the relationship between self-concept, self-esteem and behaviour, one could reasonably postulate that a nurse would be motivated to adopt a professional role that fulfils their expectations of the role, and thus serves to promote positive self-esteem and self-concept. The ways in which nurses regard and thus perform their roles will therefore be individual and essentially different.

In summary

Recent central and local government publications have drawn attention to the specific contribution of the registered nurse in the provision of care for older adults. However, there has been no definition of what constitutes the registered nurse role.

The literature suggests that patients and nurses may have different expectations of the registered nursing role. It may be that the patient's perceptions are shaped either by the aspects of care that are important to them, or by their general expectations of state healthcare provision. The nurse's perception may be motivated either by a professional endeavour to elevate the status of nursing, or by a personal desire to achieve a positive professional self-concept.

Although some suggestions have been made, the extent of the differences in the way in which nurses and non-nurses perceive the registered nurse's role in relation to caring for older adults is not known. Without this knowledge, it is not possible to evaluate the potential effect of such perceptual differences on the assessment and fulfilment of an individual's registered nursing care needs.

Key points

- Nurses need to be aware that their perceptions of the registered nurse's role may differ from those of other nurses.
- Nurses should appreciate that there may be differences in how they and their patients perceive the nurse's role, and that this may result in differences in expectations of the care that nurses deliver.
- These differences may influence individual patients' and nurses' expectations of nursing care, and thus the way in which they approach the assessment process.

References

1 Department of Health (2001) *National Service Framework for Older People.* Department of Health, London.
2 Department of Health (2001) *Health and Social Care Act.* The Stationery Office, London.
3 Department of Health (2001) *The Single Assessment Process: consultation papers and process.* Department of Health, London.
4 Department of Health (2001) *Fair Access to Care Services: consultation draft.* Department of Health, London.
5 Department of Health (2001) *NHS Funded Nursing Care. Practice guide and workbook.* Department of Health, London.
6 The Health Service Ombudsman (2003) *NHS Funding for Long-Term Care.* The Stationery Office, London.
7 Department of Health (2001) *Care Homes for Older People: national minimum standards.* The Stationery Office, London.
8 Taylor H (2003) *An examination of the perceived role of the nurse providing care for older adults.* Proceedings of the Fourth Annual Research Conference of the School of Nursing and Midwifery Studies and Associated Hospitals, Trinity College Dublin, November 2003.
9 Royal Commission on Long-Term Care (1999) *With Respect to Old Age: long-term care – rights and responsibilities.* The Stationery Office, London.
10 Nursing and Midwifery Council (2004) *The NMC Code of Professional Conduct: standards for conduct, performance and ethics.* Nursing and Midwifery Council, London.

11 Royal College of Nursing (2002) *Defining Nursing*. Royal College of Nursing, London.

12 Royal College of Nursing (2002) *Behind the Headlines: a review of the UK nursing labour market in 2001*. Royal College of Nursing, London.

13 Royal College of Nursing (1997) *Royal College of Nursing Assessment Tool for Nursing Older People*. Royal College of Nursing, London.

14 Jones JA (1988) Clinical reasoning in nursing. *J Adv Nurs.* **13:** 185–92.

15 Robinson A and Street A (2004) Improving networks between acute care nurses and an aged care assessment team. *J Clin Nurs.* **13:** 486–96.

16 Milne HA and McWilliam CL (1996) Considering nursing resource as 'caring time.' *J Adv Nurs.* **23:** 810–19.

17 Hudson KA and Sexton DL (1996) Perceptions about nursing care: comparing elders' and nurses' priorities. *J Gerontol Nurs.* **22** (12): 41–6.

18 Bowers BJ, Fibich B and Jacobson N (2001) Care-as-service, care-as-relating, care-as-comfort: understanding nursing home residents' definitions of quality. *Gerontologist.* **41:** 539–45.

19 Brykczynska G (1993) Nursing values: nightmares and nonsense. In: M Joelley and G Brykzynska (eds) *Nursing: its hidden agendas*. Edward Arnold, London.

20 Banks S (2001) *Ethics and Values in Social Work*. Palgrave, Basingstoke.

21 Schon D (1987) *Educating the Reflective Practitioner: towards a new design for teaching and learning in the profession*. Jossey-Bass, San Francisco, CA.

22 Ajzen I and Fishbein M (1980) *Understanding Attitudes and Predicting Social Behaviour*. Prentice-Hall Inc., Englewood Cliffs, NJ.

23 Arthur D (1992) Measuring the professional self-concept of nurses: a critical review. *J Adv Nurs.* **17:** 712–19.

24 Burns RB (1979) *The Self-Concept in Theory, Measurement, Development and Behaviour*. Longman, Harlow.

25 Strein W (1993) Advances in research on academic self-concept: implications for school psychology. *School Psychol Rev.* **22:** 273–84.

26 Elliott G (2000) *'Teach Granny too.' Images of ageing: towards a contemporary theory of lifespan development*. Paper presented at the British Educational Research Association Conference, University of Cardiff, 7–10 September 2000.

27 Rosenberg M (1979) *Conceiving the Self*. Basic Books, New York.

28 Goodman N (2001) Failure of the dream: notes for a research program on self-esteem and failed identity in adulthood. In: TJ Owens, S Stryker and N Goodman (eds) *Extending Self-Esteem Theory and Research*. Cambridge University Press, Cambridge.

29 Ervin LH and Stryker S (2001) Theorizing the relationship between self-esteem and identity. In: TJ Owens, S Stryker and N Goodman (eds) *Extending Self-Esteem Theory and Research*. Cambridge University Press, Cambridge.

30 Phillips S (1996) Labouring the emotions: expanding the remit of nursing work? *J Adv Nurs.* **24:** 139–43.

31 Barnard A and Sandelowski M (2001) Technology and humane nursing care: (ir)reconcilable or invented difference? *J Adv Nurs.* **34:** 356–66.

32 Ellul J (1990) *The Technological Bluff*. Eerdsmans Publishing Company, Grand Rapids, MI.

33 Aggleton P and Chalmers H (2000) *Nursing Models and Nursing Practice* (2e). Macmillan, Basingstoke.

34 Liss P-E (1998) Assessing health care need: the conceptual foundation. In: S Baldwin (ed.) *Needs Assessment and Community Care: clinical practice and policy making*. Butterworth-Heinemann, Oxford.

35 Sheaff R (1996) *The Need for Healthcare*. Routledge, London.

36 Baltes MM (1996) *The Many Faces of Dependency in Old Age*. Cambridge University Press, Cambridge.

37 Lockwood A and Marshall M (1999) Can a standardised needs assessment be used to

improve the care of people with severe mental disorders? A pilot study of 'needs feedback'. *J Adv Nurs.* **30:** 1408–15.

38 Peplau H (1988) *Interpersonal Relations in Nursing.* Macmillan, London.

39 Neuman B (1995) *The Neuman Systems Model.* Appleton and Lange, Norwalk, CT.

40 Chang AM and Twinn S (1995) Role determination in nursing – implications for service provision. *J Nurs Manag.* **3:** 25–34.

41 Challis D *et al.* (2004) The value of specialist clinical assessment of older people prior to entry to care homes. *Age Ageing,* **33:** 25–34.

42 Reid J (2004) *Secretary of State for Health – Dr John Reid*; www.number-10.gov.uk/ouput/Page1388.asp (accessed 30/03/04).

43 Summerfield C and Babb P (eds) (2003) *Social Trends 33.* The Stationery Office, London.

44 Taylor H (2005) *The nursing assessment of older adults.* PhD thesis (unpublished), University College Worcester.

45 Thompson JE and Thompson HO (1990) Values: directional signals for life choices. *Neonatal Network.* **8:** 83–94.

Chapter 4

The role of decisions and judgements as part of the assessment process

Chapter 2 explored the concept of nursing assessment. It established that this process involves the nurse identifying a patient's nursing care needs, and thus their requirement for nursing interventions. An assessment may focus on one aspect of need (e.g. their cognitive status using the Mini-Mental State Examination[1]), or it may consider the whole patient and their biological, sociological and psychological needs.[2]

A reliable assessment of a patient's condition is clearly important if they are to receive care that is appropriate to their needs. This chapter describes how assessment involves the nurse making decisions and judgements about the patient, their abilities and their health status. Two disparate theoretical perspectives on decision making are explored, namely *intuition theory* and the *information-processing model*. A third alternative is offered – the *cognitive-continuum theory*, and it is suggested that this provides a theoretical compromise between these two paradigms. Finally, it is established that the reliability of an assessment will depend on the accuracy and reliability of these decisions and judgements.

What are decisions and judgements?

Various terms have been used in the literature to describe judgement and decision making, including 'clinical judgement'[3] and 'clinical decision making'.[4] Dowie[5] defines clinical judgements as 'the assessment of alternatives', whereas a decision is defined as 'choosing between alternatives' (p. 8). Thompson and Dowding[6] further relate these terms by describing 'clinical judgement' as the process and 'clinical decision making' as the outcome (p. 8). Cioffi[7] regards judgements as the basis of clinical decisions. She uses the analogy of judgement being equivalent to a medical diagnosis, whereas a decision is the evaluation and selection of the most appropriate treatment. Judgements involve an evaluation of information about a patient. Allied with this evaluation is the making of predictions (e.g. on the basis of what is known about this patient's ability to mobilise, how likely is it that they will fall over?).[7]

The distinction that Cioffi[7] makes between judgements and decisions echoes that of Crow *et al.*[8] Research by the latter suggests that although the intended outcomes may be different, there are similarities in the cognitive processes used in medical diagnosis and nursing assessment,[8] with both operationalising a 'directed information search' (p. 211). They describe the aim of 'medical diagnosis' as being to 'establish an explanation for the patient's presenting problem', whereas in a 'nursing assessment . . .the aim appears to be to provide an accurate picture of the patient's current condition or situation' (p. 206).

This research[8] also indicates that there are parallels between clinical diagnosis and nursing assessment. Both require an informed and organised search for information, motivated by cognitive processes and involving both decisions and judgements. Inherent to this is the seeking of new information and the assimilation of existing knowledge in an attempt to determine the patient's health status. Nurses will formulate a number of judgements in the process of their assessment of a patient, which will then provide a basis for their clinical decisions.

How are decisions and judgements made?

Judgement and decision-making theory have been the subject of investigation by researchers in nursing and other healthcare disciplines.[9–11] Efforts have been made to gain insight into how people make these decisions.[9, 11–13]

Information-processing theory

Thompson and Dowding[6] describe information processing as being one of the most influential models of decision making adopted by researchers in the health professions. Although much of this work centres on the work of doctors and the making of clinical diagnoses,[13] variations of the information-processing model have been widely adopted in nurse decision-making research.[10,14,15]

The basis of information-processing theory is the research of Newell and Simon.[16] They endeavoured to understand how the human mind works when it is processing information. On the basis of their findings they propose that there are limits to human short-term memory. This means that when making decisions there is no capacity to deal with all the complex information from various sources that may be pertinent to the situation. This will result in the need to make representations of the problem on the basis of carefully selected information – what Elstein and Bordage[13] describe as 'schematised portrayals' (p. 110). These will not provide a complete and exhaustive range of possibilities, but they do offer a basis for decision making. The nurse, faced with information that provokes the need to make a decision, will not have the cognitive capacity to deal with all of the necessary information in one attempt. They will therefore, in the face of their interpretation of the situation, break it down into a small number of initial hypotheses. Typical examples might be 'If X were true, what would I expect to see?' or 'If this patient was having a CVA, what signs and symptoms would I expect to see?'. This will guide the retrieval of information from memories of similar situations. Thus the data collection is guided until the nurse is able to make a decision. Elstein and Bordage[13] have described four stages to this process.

1 Cue acquisition occurs. This is a preliminary gathering of data about the patient (before or after the patient encounter), either from observation or from sources such as diagnostic tests.
2 Hypotheses are generated on the basis of information obtained from observations of the patient and retrieved from the nurse's memory.
3 Cue interpretation occurs, whereby the nurse uses the hypotheses that have

been generated to evaluate the available information and ascertain whether it supports the hypotheses.

4 Hypothesis evaluation occurs, whereby the nurse decides whether, in the face of the combined data available, any of the hypotheses can be verified. If they are unable to do this, they will proceed through the cycle again, collecting more data and generating additional hypotheses until they are in the position to verify a hypothesis.

Consider the following example.

- *Cue acquisition*: A patient suddenly and loudly complains to their nurse that they have a pain in their head. The nurse sits down with the patient and asks if there is anything else wrong. The patient rubs at their face and tells the nurse that it 'feels funny'. Their speech appears slurred.
- *Hypothesis generation*: The nurse is aware that this pain is new, and the patient is clearly 'not right'. The nurse's initial thoughts are that the patient is simply suffering from a headache and is generally unwell; that they have neuralgia or that they are having a cerebrovascular accident.
- *Cue interpretation*: The patient has a severe headache of sudden onset. They also have slurred speech and facial numbness. These are known symptoms of cerebrovascular accident.
- *Hypothesis evaluation*: The patient now appears confused, and their speech is even more slurred. This certainly seems to be more than just a headache or neuralgia, and the nurse concludes that their third hypothesis is correct and that their patient is experiencing a cerebrovascular accident.

This entire process could take only moments, and it is possible that the nurse could be entirely unaware that their brain was busily collecting data and generating and then either accepting or rejecting hypotheses. On the other hand, they might be acutely aware of what was going on, and actively seek further information, by checking the patient's blood pressure or assessing their level of consciousness. They might quickly come to a conclusion, or become mystified when they could not verify a hypothesis to explain their observations.

The role of intuition

Some nurse theorists have expressed their lack of satisfaction with the information-processing model of decision making. They include Marks-Maran,[17] who proposed that a quest to establish a professional identity has motivated nurse theorists to operate within what she considers to be a positivist paradigm. She suggests that this might be considered to have a higher status than knowledge based on less easily quantified measures. The adoption of information-processing models of decision making and the dismissal of the role of intuition was an example offered by Marks-Maran[17] of such a theoretical shift.

'Intuition' is defined by Benner *et al.*[9] as 'a judgement without rationale, a direct apprehension and response to calculative rationality' (p. 8). They suggest that intuition is a skill developed through experience and that it plays a significant role in the practice of expert nurses. Thompson and Dowding[6] explored the concept of intuition and found vagaries in the way in which it was perceived and described by nurse theorists. Common themes were that intuition is an unexplained, spontaneous and irrational process of thinking born of expertise. They also asserted the difficulties that nurses experience in the articulation of intuitive models of thinking.[6] This difficulty could account for Marks-Maran's[17] suggestion that the role of intuition as a means of explaining the way in which nurses make decisions has traditionally been underplayed.

Conversely, Thompson and Dowding[6] believe that the role of intuition as a means of explaining decision making and judgements in nursing has become influential. It is possible that this is a reaction against positivism. Indeed, Benner et al.[9] are dismissive of the 'disengaged, scientific or theoretical reasoning promoted by cognitive theorists' (p. 1) within the nursing context. They regard the relationship of the practitioner in rational models as being 'outside the situation, touching reality only through mental representations' (p. 8). This is quite unlike intuition, which requires the practitioner's involvement with the patient, their story and the way that illness has affected them, viewed in the context of the nurse's own clinical experience and expertise. They argue that, to some extent, every human experience will be influenced by the way in which that individual's mind interprets it in relation to their existing knowledge and previous experiences. They regard the cognitivist approach as separating the emotional component of decision making into the affective aspect and the cognitive appraisal of this. Somewhat confusingly, however, they report how expert nurses use rationality as a means of checking intuitions. They suggest that nurses evaluate the consequences should an intuition be wrong, and that they may assess the 'relevance and adequacy of past experiences that may underlie a current intuition' (p. 11). It is difficult to see how the irrational basis of intuition can be asserted within such a context and indeed, they agree that there may be some place for rationality: [9]

> Calculative reasoning, requiring analysis of particular situations, consulting research and theoretical literature for possible interpretations and solutions, and explicit weighing of the possible outcomes and consequences of each potential action, does and should figure prominently in the practice of experienced clinicians. (p. 12)

Easen and Wilcockson[18] agree that the dichotomy between intuition and rational decision making in nursing may be false. They performed a detailed analysis of the various contributors to writings on intuition, and suggest that 'some of the confusion associated with this concept [intuition] seems to stem from the belief that intuition is an irrational process'. As a consequence, it is assumed that intuition can be neither fully understood nor explained. The authors propose that 'by the standards of reasoning held by western society, intuition is an irrational process but with a rational basis', because for something to be considered rational, it must be achieved by means of a process that is 'conscious, systematic and explicable' (p. 672).

Easen and Wilcockson[18] justify the rational basis by describing fundamental elements of intuition. The first such element is the need for the practitioner to be able to recognise patterns in the new experience and to associate them with those from past experiences stored within their knowledge base. As practitioners become more adept at the work that they do, they will become less aware of their patterns of action, they will need to think about them less and their performance will seem to occur without any kind of conscious thinking. An intuitive act is rapid and performed in response to the recognition of specific indicators. This will be without any conscious recognition of the process. Furthermore, they suggest that 'intuitive thinking has certain essential features and involves the use of a sound, rational, relevant knowledge base in situations that, through experience, are so familiar that the person has learned how to recognise and act on the appropriate patterns' (p. 667).

Cognitive continuum theory

Thompson[19] and Harbison[20] both argue that a rigid adherence to either information-processing theory or intuition fails to adequately explain decision making observed in nursing. They suggest that the cognitive continuum theory[21] acknowledges the complex interplay of both rational thinking and intuitive processes in decision making. This was used by Hamm[21] as a way of explaining that the decision-making processes utilised in any situation will depend on the context and complexity of that situation – that 'there are different modes of cognition, analysis and intuition' (p. 101). The mode of cognition would range from intuition to analysis, depending on the nature of the decision-making task. A highly structured task with plenty of time available would evoke a decision based on analysis. Conversely, an ill-structured task requiring a rapid response might result in an intuitive decision.

Thompson[19,22] and Harbison[20] identify the cognitive continuum as providing a useful middle ground between the systemic–positivistic and intuitive–humanistic paradigms, permitting nurse theorists to acknowledge the contribution of theoretical input from other disciplines,[20] indicating a kind of philosophical 'sitting on the fence'.

Investigating how nurses make decisions

Research conducted by Corcoran[15] used verbal protocols to investigate the decision-making process in planning care in three simulated cases of varying complexity. The findings indicate that expert nurses (i.e. those nurses with a greater knowledge and experience of their work role) adopted a broader planning approach to decision making, which was based on a breadth of observations and knowledge. No such pattern was obvious for the less experienced nurses in their sample, who tended to focus on more narrow approaches, contemplating one factor or observation at a time. In non-complex cases, the experienced nurses used a systematic approach, working on the basis of what was familiar and what they had encountered before. With complex cases the approach was more opportunistic, a method adopted by novice nurses regardless of the complexity of the task.

Although Corcoran's study[15] was conducted on a small sample consisting of six 'expert' and five 'novice' nurses, the results are broadly echoed by those of Tanner et al.[11] Their findings from a larger sample of 43 nurses indicate that more accurate diagnosis and more systematic data collection are associated with greater levels of nurse knowledge and experience. Like Corcoran's study,[15] this research again used simulated situations and verbal protocols. Taking these findings together, there is some indication that more experienced nurses are able to adapt their decision making according to the complexity of the task and their familiarity with the situation.

The research of Thompson et al.[23] and a number of the other studies focus on what might be categorised as 'technical nursing care'. In the study by Thompson et al.,[23] data were obtained from a convenience sample of 122 nurses working in three large acute hospitals in the north of England. The nurses were asked to think of a clinical question that they either had made or might make in their clinical practice. They were provided with some example questions to guide them, which included selecting the best time to start cardiac rehabilitation subsequent to myocardial infarction, deciding which method of blood monitoring was likely to be best in a young adult with moderate learning difficulties, and answering patient questions about the risks of cerebrovascular accident associated with thrombolytic treatment.[23]

It could be said that the example questions directed the nurses to think about the technical aspects of acute care. Although the authors do acknowledge that the study examined only nurses working in the acute care sector, it could be argued that the results would have wider applicability had the nurses (all of whom were working on acute medical, surgical and coronary care wards) not been specifically directed to think about decisions based on these 'technical' aspects of their clinical role, rather than the more 'hands-on' caring or staff supervision described in Chapter 3.

This reflects a number of other studies of clinical decision making – for example, calling medical emergency teams to patients,[24] an acute renal problem,[25] the presentation of three simulated patients either in need of or in receipt of acute care,[11] and the treatment of pressure sores.[26] A further study by Botti and Reeve[10] investigated the diagnostic reasoning ability of 60 third-year and second-year students when they were faced with six simulated clinical problems of varying complexity. The problems were not defined in the paper, but were constructed using the medical surgical textbooks and undergraduate curriculum being studied by the students, and so were likely to have focused on the provision of acute care. Even in the study conducted by Benner et al.,[9] the sample was asked to provide a narrative detailing an aspect of their practice in the field of what the researchers termed 'critical care'. These studies are unlikely to entirely reflect the work done by nurses caring for older adults. It is important that those reviewing research findings in the area of nurse decision making are aware of these methodological issues relating to nurse decision-making research.

A study conducted by Manias et al.[27] was unusual in that it investigated the decision-making activities of a group of 12 volunteer graduate nurses actually at work in an Australian hospital. Their decisions were observed as they took place in the field, rather than by using clinical simulations. The nurses were surveyed as they administered drugs, and were asked questions in order to clarify and explain their decisions. Analysis of the interview transcripts indicated that the most frequently used decision-making model was hypothetico-deductive (information processing). However, the researchers acknowledge that the behaviour of the nurses may have been influenced by the knowledge that they were being observed. It would appear that any method of investigating decision making will be subject to its own specific limitations.

Expertise in nursing

The terms 'expert nurse' and 'novice nurse' have already been used in this chapter. At this point an exploration of the concept and definition of 'expertise' in nursing is felt to be necessary. Expertise has been identified as a prerequisite for skilled and accurate decision making, whether cognitive or intuitive.[15,28,29] However, there is no consensus as to what actually constitutes an 'expert nurse'. Although Benner[28] offers no prescription of the time taken for a nurse to make the transition from novice to expert, for other researchers this has not been the case. For example, Corcoran[15] has compared the decision making of expert and novice nurses. Her selection criteria for an expert nurse were that they had to be a registered nurse, currently engaged in a position of leadership with at least 18 months' experience of working in the specialty in conjunction with one other of the following: a published article in that field, having made presentations in that area of expertise or having offered continuing education in that field. The novice nurses would be registered nurses working as staff nurses with less than six months' experience in the field.[15]

Cioffi's descriptive study[29] was based on a sample of 20 volunteers. Within this group, 'experienced nurses' were deemed to be those with at least five years' experience in the specialty, and the 'less experienced' had between one and two years' experience. Although the time spans are different, both of these relate domain-specific knowledge to expertise. This view is further expounded by Benner et al.[9] who, although not associating any time span with the concept of 'expertise' (i.e. 'once you have been in this role for X years, you can consider yourself an expert'), suggest that 'there are, perhaps, no expert nurses, but certainly many nurses achieve expertise in the areas of their specialisation' (p. 36). Lamond and Farnell[26] adopted 'peer evaluation' as a determinant of expertise. In their convenience sample of seven 'expert' and seven 'novice' nurses, the expert nurses were those considered by their managers to be 'experts' in practice.

It is clear, therefore, that researchers do not uniformly define the concept of expertise in nursing. Some caution should therefore be exercised when comparing the findings of studies that make reference to 'expert nurses' and 'novice nurses'.

In summary

In this chapter, two distinct perspectives on decision-making theory have been considered, namely information processing and the intuitive decision as advocated by Benner et al.[9] However, it is argued that a rigid adherence either to intuition theory or to information processing as based on the logical cognitive scientific modelling of Newell and Simon[16] fails to adequately explain the decision making that is observed in clinical situations.[19,20] The cognitive continuum theory provides a useful alternative perspective.

However, regardless of the paradigm adopted to explain decision making in nursing, a need for both acquired and stored knowledge and information cannot be disputed. Judgement and decisions have been established as inherent to the assessment process. Whenever nurses are required to make decisions or judgements about their patient, these will be based on some knowledge or cues, even if the decision appears to be intuitive.

Chapters 5 and 6 will investigate sources of information that nurses may use as part of the decision-making process, and will discuss how the reliability of that information may influence the accuracy of the assessment.

Key points

- Making decisions and judgements is inherent to the assessment process.
- There are a number of theories explaining how decisions and judgements are made.
- Regardless of the theory adopted, these decisions and judgements will be based on acquired information of some kind.

References

1 Folstein M, Folstein S and McHugh PR (1975) Mini-Mental State: a practical method for grading the cognitive state of patients for the clinician. *J Psychiatr Res.* **12**: 189–98.

2 Department of Health (2002) *The Single Assessment Process: assessment tools and scales*; www.doh.gov.uk/scg/sap/toolsandscales (accessed 12/12/02).

3 Dowding D and Thompson C (2003) Measuring the quality of judgement and decision-making in nursing. *J Adv Nurs.* **44**: 49–57.

4 Dowie J and Elstein A (1988) *Professional Judgement. A reader in clinical decision making.* Cambridge University Press, Cambridge.

5 Dowie J (1993) Clinical decision analysis: background and introduction. In: H Llewelyn and A Hopkins (eds) *Analysing How We Reach Clinical Decisions.* Royal College of Physicians, London.

6 Thompson C and Dowding D (2002) Decision making and judgement in nursing – an introduction. In: C Thompson and D Dowding (eds) *Clinical Decision Making and Judgement in Nursing.* Churchill Livingstone, Edinburgh.

7 Cioffi J (2002) What are clinical judgements? In: C Thompson and D Dowding (eds) *Clinical Decision Making and Judgement in Nursing.* Churchill Livingstone, Edinburgh.

8 Crow RA, Chase J and Lamond D (1995) The cognitive component of nursing assessment: an analysis. *J Adv Nurs.* **22**: 206–12.

9 Benner P, Tanner CA, and Chesla CA (1996) *Expertise in Nursing Practice: caring, clinical judgement and ethics.* Springer Publishing Company, New York.

10 Botti M and Reeve R (2002) Role of knowledge and ability in student nurses' clinical decision-making. *Nurs Health Sci.* **5**: 39–49.

11 Tanner CA *et al.* (1987) Diagnostic reasoning strategies of nurses and nursing students. *Nurs Res.* **36**: 358–63.

12 Benner P, Hooper-Kyriakidis P and Stannard D (1999) *Clinical Wisdom in Critical Care: a thinking in action approach.* WB Saunders Company, Philadelphia, PA.

13 Elstein AS and Bordage G (1988) Psychology and clinical reasoning. In: J Dowie and A Elstein (eds) *Professional Judgement: a reader in clinical decision making.* Cambridge University Press, Cambridge.

14 Bryans A and McIntosh J (1996) Decision making in community nursing: an analysis of the stages of decision making as they relate to community nursing assessment practice. *J Adv Nurs.* **24**: 24–30.

15 Corcoran S (1986) Task complexity and nursing expertise as factors in decision making. *Nurs Res.* **35**: 107–12.

16 Newell A and Simon HA (1972) *Human Problem Solving.* Prentice Hall, Englewood Cliffs, NJ.

17 Marks-Maran D (1997) Intuition: 'just knowing' in nursing. In: D Marks-Maran and P Rose (eds) *Reconstructing Nursing: beyond art and science.* Baillière Tindall, London.

18 Easen P and Wilcockson J (1996) Intuition and rational decision making in professional thinking: a false dichotomy? *J Adv Nurs.* **24:** 667–73.

19 Thompson C (1999) A conceptual treadmill: the need for 'middle ground' in clinical decision-making theory in nursing. *J Adv Nurs.* **30:** 1222–9.

20 Harbison J (2001) Clinical decision-making in nursing: theoretical perspectives and their relevance to practice. *J Adv Nurs.* **35:** 126–33.

21 Hamm RM (1988) Clinical intuition and clinical analysis: expertise and the cognitive continuum. In: J Dowie and A Elstein (eds) *Professional Judgement: a reader in clinical decision making.* Cambridge University Press, Cambridge.

22 Thompson C (2002) Human error, bias, decision making and judgement in nursing – the need for a systematic approach. In: C Thompson and D Dowding (eds) *Clinical Decision Making and Judgement in Nursing.* Churchill Livingstone, Edinburgh.

23 Thompson C *et al.* (2001) Research information in nurses' clinical decision making: what is useful? *J Adv Nurs.* **36:** 376–88.

24 Cioffi J (2000) Nurses' experiences of making decisions to call emergency assistance to their patients. *J Adv Nurs.* **32:** 108–14.

25 Cholowski KM and Chan LKS (1992) Diagnostic reasoning among second-year nursing students. *J Adv Nurs.* **17:** 1171–81.

26 Lamond D and Farnell S (1998) The treatment of pressure sores: a comparison of novice and expert nurses' knowledge, information use and decision accuracy. *J Adv Nurs.* **27:** 280–6.

27 Manias E, Aitken R and Dunning T (2004) Decision-making models used by 'graduate nurses' managing patients' medications. *J Adv Nurs.* **47:** 270–8.

28 Benner P (1984) *From Novice to Expert: excellence and power in clinical nursing practice.* Addison-Wesley, Menlo Park, CA.

29 Cioffi J (1998) Decision making by emergency nurses in triage assessments. *Accid Emerg Nurs.* **6:** 184–91.

Chapter 5

Making an accurate assessment

Research conducted by Lamond[1] supports the idea that judgements help the nurse to establish a description of the patient's status or change in status. It has already been demonstrated in Chapter 4 that in order for a nurse to make judgements and decisions as part of the assessment process, they first need to gather and process information from a variety of sources. The complex nature of the decision-making process has also been explored, and involves a number of variables, including task complexity, nurse expertise, selection of information, sources of information and urgency of decision.

The need for a reliable assessment of a patient's requirement for nursing interventions has been established (*see* Chapter 2). Without this assessment it will not be possible for the individual's needs to be addressed appropriately. Judgements and decisions are inherent to the assessment process (*see* Chapter 4). It is clear, therefore, that if an assessment is to be reliable then the judgements and decisions, and the information underpinning them, must also be reliable. This chapter investigates factors that may render an assessment unreliable. First, however, it is necessary to establish the concept of accuracy in judgement and decision making.

How accurate are judgements and decisions?

It has been indicated that evaluation of the accuracy of judgements and decisions made in practice is difficult,[2] there being no established definition of what constitutes an 'accurate' decision or judgement in nursing.[3] Thompson[3] has explored a number of possible definitions of an accurate decision, including a decision which results in an outcome which most nurses would arrive at, one that is based on the most reliable and valid supporting evidence, and finally that which best addresses the available human and material resources.

Other researchers have also made an attempt to define accuracy. For example, Botti and Reeve[4] investigated the decision-making ability of student nurses and define an accurate decision as one that corresponded with that predetermined by the researchers. This definition of accuracy was also applied in research conducted by Corcoran.[5] Lamond and Farnell[6] did not specify how they had defined accuracy in their comparison of knowledge, information use and decision accuracy between novice and expert nurses. However, they did state that the decisions made by their convenience sample of seven expert and seven novice nurses would be compared with the gold standard decisions made by a panel of experts in the field of pressure sores. This implies that in this study, like those of Corcoran[5] and Botti and Reeve,[4] an accurate decision was one closely allied to that which would be made by expert nurses, based on the application of expertise and knowledge to the information available. This suggests that validation of expertise can only be conveyed by an expert, echoing the assertion by Benner[7] that only an expert judge can determine whether a nurse has reached a level of expertise in their practice. Difficulties in defining expertise (*see* Chapter 4) would further complicate the issue of defining decision accuracy.

It would appear that there is some variation in use, but the concept of accurate decisions or judgements is used frequently in this book. A consideration of the literature suggests that an accurate decision or judgement will be one that, in the face of the evidence available, corresponds most closely with the consensus of expert opinion. It will also be justifiable and have internal consistency.[8] In other words, the decision appears to correlate with all the other available evidence, and is not contradicted or challenged by other decisions or judgements made by the nurse.

Errors in judgement

Having considered the issues of accuracy in judgement and decision making, it is acknowledged that some decisions and judgements will be inaccurate, for a variety of reasons that are often more complicated than simply a fault in information processing.[9] For example, the development of expert knowledge in a specific field is generally viewed as having a beneficial effect on decision making, yet it could be argued that such practice-specific knowledge, cognitive information gathering and organisational strategies may result in inflexible approaches to decision making.[10] For example, nurses working on a medical ward are unlikely to have the practice-specific knowledge necessary to make decisions on an intensive therapy unit. Nurses without knowledge of and expertise in the care of older adults may lack the practice-specific knowledge necessary to make effective decisions about those patients' needs and care (*see* Chapter 2). Different nurses may perceive cues and observations in disparate ways. Indeed, social judgement theory suggests that observations and cues can be weighted in different ways by the clinician during hypothesis formulation, depending on how they perceive the patient and the observational cues.[11]

If a nursing assessment of an older adult is to be accurate, then the judgements and decisions made as part of the assessment process must be accurate.[1] This will be determined by the way in which information is obtained,[9] and how observational cues are recognised and weighted by the nurse.[11] Accuracy will also be determined by the quality of the information available to the nurse (*see* Chapter 4). There are therefore two main potential sources of error in the assessment process – those associated with the nurse him- or herself, and those external to the nurse. External factors will incorporate any provider of information contributing to judgements and decisions made during the assessment process, including the patient him- or herself, his or her relatives and other healthcare professionals.[11] These two sources of potential error will each be considered in turn.

Sources of error related to the nurse

When making a comprehensive assessment of a patient using an assessment tool such as the Royal College of Nursing Assessment Tool for Nursing Older People,[12] it is unlikely that all judgements made by the nurse will be in specific response to immediate and observable changes in the patient's condition. They are more likely to represent a complex combination of judgements and decisions, like those in the simulated scenarios used in research by Corcoran[6] and Tanner et al.,[13] for example (see Chapter 4).

So where might this information come from? Lamond[1] conducted an investigation that compared the patient information given in patient notes and charts with that provided during shift handover reports. The study was based on a convenience sample of 20 shift reports (10 reports from surgical wards and 10 reports from medical wards) from four wards situated within two general hospitals in northern England. Content analysis was performed on the notes and charts of a random sample of 60 of the patients reported. Lamond[1] describes the coding scheme that she used during her investigation, based on the information sources identified during an earlier investigation with which she had been involved,[10] and included both objective and subjective measures, and what she termed 'global judgements'. These were considered to be 'evaluations made by the nurses that were non-specific in nature' (p. 797). An example of a global judgement was identified (*'they are a bit better today'*). Specific categories of information were described as general information (e.g. name, age and diagnosis), physical information (e.g. appearance, 'care needs', diet), physical measures (e.g. pulse, blood tests, Waterlow score), functional information (e.g. sleeping, drinking), psychological information (e.g. 'self-management', 'verbal response', confusion), social information (e.g. occupation, 'home facilities', next of kin), family information (e.g. ability to visit, understanding), nursing interventions (e.g. 'patient care needs'), medical treatment, global judgements and management issues.

Other research undertaken by Lamond et al.[14] involved conducting a semi-structured interview in which a convenience sample consisting of 104 nurses was asked to talk about decisions that they had made during one nursing shift. Four types of judgement and their associated information sources were identified, with judgements most frequently utilised being 'descriptive' and 'evaluative'. The judgement types were summarised as follows:[9]

- *causal judgements (diagnosis)* – explaining a problem by using a statement of patient status which has been based on specific characteristics
- *descriptive judgements* – the use of a statement of patient status describing specific characteristics, which is either based directly on the nurse's observations or derived elsewhere
- *evaluative judgements* – the use of a statement of a change in patient status describing specific characteristics, which is either based directly on the nurse's observations or derived elsewhere
- *inference judgements* – the use of a statement of patient status describing specific characteristics, which has not been based on any information concerning the patient from any source.

(p. 49)

The findings of Lamond et al.[15] indicate that when making decisions about patient care and ward management, nurses relied heavily on verbal information obtained from other staff and the patient (41.3% of information sources used). Observations of the patient, their family and other staff were also widely used (21.3%), as was information obtained from written records (16.5%). These findings indicate that the nurse would be required to recall and sift through a diverse range of information about the patient, including the observations that they themselves have made about the patient, information that they have read, and information that they have been told by other members of staff. They will also have been given information by the patient him- or herself and by the patient's family and friends.[16] There will be some information that they have read in journals and books.[17] This list is not exhaustive, and these sources of information will be explored in more detail in Chapter 6.

The role of the nurse's memory

Findings such as those of Cioffi[9] indicate that decisions are often based on a nurse's recalled observations of their patient. It is therefore important to consider the role of memory in decision making. A full and detailed examination of the enormous body of literature relating to memory is beyond the scope of this book. However, a number of key points will be examined in order to provide some insight into the way in which cognitive processes may impair the recall of information and thus the efficacy of decision making. In other words, if nurses forget some important piece of information relating to their patient, it is likely that any decisions made that require this information will be less than accurate. For example, consider the scenario in Box 5.1.

Box 5.1

Mary has a patient called Jeremy, who is usually able to mobilise safely and without any support. One day, however, Mary observes Jeremy stumble. He quickly grabs on to a handrail and prevents himself from falling. Mary checks and finds that there are no obstructions which could have caused the fall. When asked, Jeremy tells Mary that he just felt a little light-headed. Mary intends to check his blood pressure and blood glucose levels, but gets called away and forgets to do this. A few days later she is completing an evaluation of Jeremy's nursing assessment. She comes to the section relating to mobility, and forgetting his stumble writes that he has 'no problems with mobilising'. A few days later Jeremy falls again, this time fracturing his femur. He is found to suffer from postural hypotension.

Mary's assessment of Jeremy's ability to mobilise was based on an incomplete recollection of relevant information, and her judgement was therefore impaired.

Baddeley[18] suggests that *interference* can inhibit memory, and may explain forgetting: 'Memory traces are disrupted or obscured by subsequent learning, in other words forgetting occurs because of interference' (p. 142). This contrasts with other theories, which suggest that forgetting occurs because memories fade. However, Baddeley reviewed the work of McGeoch and MacDonald,[19] which supports the role of interference, indicating that the level of forgetting is increased if the interfering information is similar to that remembered.[18] This may have implications for nurses' recall of their patient observations. In other words, if a nurse makes two or more observations of their patient, the more similar the observations, the more likely the nurse is to forget their initial observation. For example, they are more likely to forget the first observation in Example 1 than in Example 2 below.

Example 1

08.20 – Mary observes Peter walking from his bed to the chair and notices that he is leaning slightly to his right.

09.40 – Mary observes Peter walking from his bed to the chair and notices that he is dragging his left foot slightly.

Example 2

08.20 – Mary observes Peter brushing his hair and notices that he is experiencing difficulty raising his right arm.

09.40 – Mary observes Peter folding his pyjamas and notices that he appears more stooped than is usual for him.

Retroactive interference refers to the learning of new information that results in the forgetting of old stored information.[18] However:

> there has been much controversy as to whether forming the second association . . . actually weakens the first, or overshadows by its great strength. Whatever occurs, there is no doubt that whatever strengthens recall of one association minimises the recall of the other.
>
> (p. 148)

This gives some insight into how nurses have come to recognise the need to use aides-mémoire and visual cues to aid memory retrieval.[18] I am sure that all nurses will have watched colleagues as they have attempted to remember whether it was the left or right arm which the patient was having difficulty manipulating that morning. They will sit in handover wriggling their own arms in a reconstruction of the movements observed in their patient, and this may help to jog their memory.

Research[20] has suggested that experienced practitioners are more expert at problem solving than novice practitioners, due to their superior memory and recall of relevant information. It was also found that the experts demonstrated a more cohesive and organised approach to their information recall, making fewer errors and showing better recall of relevant information than the novices did. In addition, there was some evidence of 'confirmatory bias', with the respondents recalling more memory-based evidence in support of the selected diagnosis than was discarded, suggesting that the experts had selectively recalled some of the evidence in support of their decision.

The context in which a nurse is required to 'remember' may also affect the efficacy of their recollection, and Godden and Baddeley's review[21] of the literature indicates that both intrinsic and extrinsic contexts influence the recall of stimuli.

They describe 'extrinsic context' as the environmental conditions at the time of the event to be recalled. There is evidence that recall is enhanced if the extrinsic context is the same at both times.[21] 'Intrinsic context' is related to the stimulus and processed at the same time (e.g. the tone, pitch and volume of the voice speaking a particular phrase).[21]

Godden and Baddeley[21] reported a significant link between intrinsic context and both recall and recognition, whereas extrinsic context has only been shown to have an effect on tests using recall. However, their research indicates no link between context and recognition, with Baddeley[18] suggesting that this could be because, when testing recognition, the appearance of what he called the target is enough to stimulate recognition of whether it has been encountered before. This would negate the need for additional environmental cues.[18] For example, if the nurse had observed a patient stumble and almost fall earlier in their shift, simply seeing that patient walking around later in the day would be enough to trigger their memory of the event. This would imply that removing the nurse from the environment in which the event occurred would potentially have a deleterious effect on event recall. It is unlikely that during the course of their working day a nurse would encounter environmental changes as significant as those in Godden and Baddeley's research on a comparison between land and underwater environments.[21] However, if the nurse is required to recall their patient observations away from the noisy, possibly malodorous clinical practice area (e.g. in a quiet office away from distractions), their recollection of events observed in the field may be impaired.

There will also be limits to how much information the nurse is able to store in their short-term memory. Indeed, the findings of Ericsson et al.[22] provide some evidence to support the suggestion that the limits of short-term memory are small. They indicate that it is not possible to actually increase the working capacity of short-term memory, but only to train the mind to store the information in long-term memory by using aids such as mnemonics. However, it should be noted that there are limitations to the findings of this study, which was based entirely on one subject. The researchers selected one undergraduate who had what they considered to be an 'average' memory and intelligence, although they did not document whether there were any specific criteria for this. This student was then engaged in a series of tests for one hour each day, between three and five days each week for a period of 18 months.

On the basis of these findings, and even after considering some methodological issues, there is some indication that nurses' observations of their patients may be vulnerable to forgetting. It is simply impossible for a nurse to remember everything that they see their patient do, or how they smell or sound. Even if nurses do remember these things, it has been suggested that 'memories are malleable'[23] and vulnerable to distortion due to either forgetting or reconstruction of that memory. This is true even for what have been described as 'flashbulb memories' – that is, memories of an unusual or notable event (e.g. what you were doing when you first heard about the events of 9/11 (11 September 2001 when two hijacked planes crashed into the World Trade Centre in New York). I can quite clearly recall hearing the news as I drove from my office in Worcester to collect my two sons from school. I took them to the dentist, and then returned home where we spent most of the evening watching the terrible events being replayed on the television. I can recall telephone conversations, and the feelings that

I experienced. I feel quite certain that my memories of that day are accurate, but there is some suggestion that this might not be so.

Neath[23] suggests that there are inaccuracies in the recall of what people may consider to be photograph-like memories of what they were doing, who they were with, and so on, possibly because if memories are not evaluated instantly, details may subsequently be added to embellish the story. On recall there will be an impression that the added and/or modified details were part of the original event. This indicates that even though people have greater confidence in their recall of 'flashbulb' than other memories, this confidence may be unfounded.[23] Neath describes a 'schema' as:

> An organised knowledge structure that reflects an individual's know-ledge, experience and expectations about some aspect of the world. Information contained in a schema is usually recruited to help recall various events.   (p. 328)

It is possible that my recollections are not an accurate memory of that terrible day, with subsequent information serving to alter my memory of how I felt at that time. Rather than a concrete entity of which the recall becomes less clear, memories of events are altered over time by reconstruction and reprocessing of the event, depending on the schema being operationalised at the time of recollection.[23] It can be seen that if nurses are required to recall some observation of their patient for assessment, then such recollections may be vulnerable to distortion, inaccuracies and forgetting.

Baddeley[18] describes how he had been unable to recall a trip to the coast made with his wife before their marriage. He was able to 'conjure up' perceptions of the town, but unable to determine whether they were based on his now forgotten visit, or images derived from the media. He recalled some very vivid and different images of the town when his wife reminded him that he had sat in some seagull droppings during the visit! This indicates that it may not be possible to determine whether a nurse's recollection of some aspect of their patient's condition is true, or has been constructed as a result of being unable to remember the actual event. Paddock et al.[24] describe how a sample of engineering students demonstrated a shift from an event in their childhood that was known about but not remembered, to constructing it as an actual memory, The students confabulated experiences and feelings after one 15-minute guided visualisation technique. This supports the suggestion that, with prompting, people are able to construct non-existent memories.

There is also evidence that memories are vulnerable to 'suggestibility',[25] with leading evidence distorting the recall of the event. An example of this would be if a nurse was specifically asked how many times a patient had experienced episodes of incontinence that day, and this then induced recollections of episodes that did not actually occur. It could even be said that the wording of descriptors in assessment tools might have a suggestive effect on the nurse's memories of that patient, evoking recollections which would not have been made if the nurse had not been asked that question. For example, if a nurse is asked whether a patient has ever demonstrated aggressive behaviour, they might think, 'Well, now you come to mention it . . . the other day, he did get a bit upset. Was that aggression? I suppose it could be in a way'.

Suggestibility has been shown to influence the reconstructive accuracy of events in eyewitness accounts.[18,23,26] This possibility is taken very seriously by the legal profession, with courts endeavouring to avoid eyewitness evidence that is thought to have been obtained by suggestible means.[27] The effect of suggestibility may be enhanced by the influential effects of interviewer behaviour,[28] or by specific characteristics of the interviewee, such as a state of anxiety, youth or low intelligence quotient.[29]

Base rate neglect

Thompson[30] cites base rate neglect as a source of error in decision making, where the individual who is making the decision ignores statistical probabilities which could preclude that decision. He cites the example of a clinician using a diagnostic test that has a high false-positive result rate for a disease with a very low level of incidence. If the clinician was to take a positive test result as evidence that the patient has the disease, they would then be ignoring the base rate. He suggests that whilst there is some (albeit what he regards as methodologically limited) evidence that nurses do use base rate recognition as a basis for their clinical decisions, there may be a tendency to ignore statistical probability when making the decisions. The nurse may focus on what may be irrelevant information.

For example, if a patient who is receiving a particular drug therapy starts to experience severe flatulence, the nurse may rationalise this by relating it to the flatulence observed in another patient who was receiving that particular drug therapy, aware that digestive problems had been cited as very rare side-effects of this medication. In this case the nurse would be neglecting the base rate by ignoring the fact that the new patient had been taking the medication for months before they experienced any problems. The medication was therefore unlikely to have been the cause of the flatulence, and any similarity to the other patient was purely coincidental. It is clear, therefore, that neglecting the base rate may contribute to errors in decision making.

The effect of the nurse's past experiences

The effects of the nurse's past experiences have been found to make a significant contribution to the decision-making process.[31] Earlier research by Cioffi[32] indicates that when making decisions about simulated patients with whom they have not had (nor will have) any actual contact, there was a higher probability of more experienced than inexperienced nurses relying on their memory of previous cases encountered. Cioffi[32] terms this the 'representativeness heuristic' (p. 189), more often operationalised with experienced nurses, who also collected fewer data than their less experienced colleagues. This is further evidence of the experienced nurses' reliance on their memories. Cioffi described these as heuristics, or 'rules of thumb' or 'subjective probability judgements'[32] (p. 185), based on work by Tversky and Kahneman.[33,34] These may also include the 'availability' heuristic, which depends on the nurse recalling a previous similar incident or case, and the 'anchoring and adjustment heuristic', where the assessment decision is made within the context of what the nurse would expect for someone who fulfilled certain criteria (e.g. 'This person is diabetic, I would expect their blood sugar level to be within such a range, but it is . . .').

The use of heuristics was found to increase in conditions where there was more uncertainty about the diagnosis.[9] There is a suggestion that nurses take short cuts in an attempt to overcome the difficulties encountered when handling a wealth of patient data, and that individuals will have their own preferred way of arriving at conclusions.[9] Cioffi[9] describes these biases as 'systematic tendencies' (p. 59), and proposes that nurses attempt to derive meaning from the presenting situation by using memorised knowledge as they 'access similar situations, cases and events or a particular example' (p. 59). For example, they might say to themselves, 'Ah, if I remember correctly, the last time Fred spiked a temperature like that he went on to get that really nasty chest infection'.

Much has been written about observational information gleaned by expert nurses from their patient, often even before that patient has demonstrated any overtly recognisable symptoms.[7,35,36] It is important to explore how this occurs in order to gain an insight into how errors may occur with such judgements. An exploration by Gardner[37] of the work of cognitive scientists such as Johnson-Laird, Kahneman and Tversky indicates that early cognitive models of human beings as logical and rational thinkers require some reconsideration. Findings suggest that people do not simply apply the same rules of logic regardless of the actual nature of the problem. Gardner[37] explains Johnson-Laird's theory of how individuals use mental models as a necessary component of syllogistic reasoning:

> One succeeds on problems to the extent that one can construct mental models that represent the relevant information in an appropriate fashion and use these mental models flexibly. . . .Logic cannot serve as a valid model of how most individuals solve most problems all of the time.   (p. 370)

This implies that individuals use their experience of the real world to construct mental models, which means that although logic may have some place in some instances, not all decisions will appear logical, or possibly rational. This has been explored in more detail in Chapter 4.

Furthermore, Gardner[37] explained how Tversky and Kahneman describe the tendency of people to be guided more by how one factor is linked with another associated factor than by the actual probability of that happening. An example of this would be if during the course of a schoolday a child is admonished by their teacher, and the teacher subsequently discovers a broken window at the school. The teacher is likely to associate this with the child whom they have told off, even though there is a low probability of that child being responsible. This depends on the person relating one experience to views that they already hold, and the way in which they frame that knowledge will influence the decisions that they make.[37] Gardner[37] states that although there had been what he termed 'philosophical criticisms' of these ideas, they do provide a useful insight into why, when given the same information, not all people would make the same decision, and indicate the need for caution when evaluating the accuracy and quality of decisions made by other people. This is because it is not possible to fully understand the complicated ways in which individuals handle the complex information with which they are presented.

With the benefit of hindsight

Thompson[38] cites 'hindsight bias' as a potential source of error at the knowledge-based level of decision making, this being the tendency people have to regard the outcome of an event or happening as having been predictable, but only once they are aware of the outcome.[39] They 'tend to view what has happened as having been inevitable' (p. 428). This would indicate that where a similar case has been encountered in the past, the nurse uses their recollected knowledge of causative links and outcomes to predict outcomes in the newly encountered case. The explanation for this process is that when reflecting on the events leading to the outcome, cognitive models are reviewed and re-evaluated. The observer will disregard information that seems irrelevant to the outcome, and emphasise that which supports it.[40] The individual's recall of the event, choice or decision will then become biased in support of the known outcome.[41]

A process model for hindsight bias, known as RAFT (Reconstruction After Feedback with Take the Best[41]), explains hindsight bias as occurring when an individual is unable to recall the choice that they made at a specified time (Time 1). They will reconstruct it at a later time (Time 3) using the same cognitive processes. However, this reconstruction relies on a recall of the information used to make the original choice, and in the face of outcome knowledge supplied at interim Time 2, this recalled knowledge and cues will be ranked in order of validity and applicability.[41] It is therefore likely that data which were not available at the time of the original choice will be retained if they are relevant, and data considered irrelevant to the choice will be discarded.[41]

Sanna et al.[40] propose that hindsight bias may encourage people to falsely believe that they had actually anticipated the outcome, thereby fostering an erroneous confidence in their decisions. There is a 'creeping determinism',[39] a post hoc perception that there could have been no other outcome. Roese and Olson[42] suggest that this implies an incompatibility or preclusion of counter-factual thinking – that the outcome was predestined. They argue that this idea adopted by some philosophers is incongruent with scientific practice,[42] and suggest a more tempered view of determinism – 'a past outcome is viewed to have been certain (i.e. "determined") only to the extent that its cause preceded it' (p. 199).

A study conducted by Reece Jones[43] used vignettes and questionnaires to investigate the reflective practice of a convenience sample of 27 nurses working in a 400-bed hospital. The findings indicate the influence of hindsight bias on nursing practice, with the researcher suggesting that this could have implications for the use of reflection on nursing practice. Indeed, one does have to question the influence of hindsight bias on reflective practice and the evaluation of what appear to be 'intuitive' decisions (i.e. those in which the nurse is believed to have made a decision about a patient before any tangible evidence has become available). For example, Cioffi[44] describes how, when reflecting on practice, 'nurses often recall experiences where patient survival has depended on skilful decision making. These decision-making situations require nurses to recognise early signs of clinical deterioration in patients' (p. 109). It could be said that if intuitive practice has been recognised, then any incidents where the nurse has not demonstrated intuition would be disregarded. For example, all of those times when the nurse failed to recognise any slight changes in condition will not be recalled, or will be discounted. If this is viewed within the context of hindsight bias, it could be said to be almost inevitable that the nurse would recognise the signs and make an effective clinical decision.

Nurses' perceptions of their patients: stereotyping and prejudice

If a nurse has stereotypical or prejudicial perceptions of a society or group, these may influence how the nurse regards individuals whom they consider to belong to that group.[45] Scrutton[46] describes ageism as a prejudicial view of older adults. It may be as apparently benign as a patronising desire to protect older people from harm, stressful events and unpleasantness, or as malignant as the overt dismissal and neglect of the needs of older people.[46] There may be a tendency to what Coupland and Coupland[47] have termed 'infantilising' older adults – to addressing them in a manner which infers that they somehow lack autonomy, or need protecting. This may arise from the perception of dependency and inability to make decisions. Ageist attitudes may influence and colour perceptions of older people and ultimately the care that they receive.[45] It is important to see beyond the physical manifestations of age if the individual's personhood is not to be denied:[48]

> The small wasted being that I am feeding is an individual who has experienced far more life than I have. They have lived through a war, maybe two. They have cooked meals, managed budgets, planted vegetables and perhaps given birth. They have known pain and hardship, joy and triumph. They have splashed through puddles in the rain and slipped on ice. (p. 70)

There is a notion that as humans we make sense of our world, or simplify it, by categorisation.[49] Hinton[49] describes how inferences about an individual are rapidly made from non-verbal information. Snap decisions or first impressions are made on the basis of an individual's physiognomy and their physique. He suggests that this association may be more significant than a fleeting impression, and that historically people have associated certain physical attributes with a person's character – the 'dizzy blonde' or the 'intellectual highbrowed egg-head'.[49]

Prototypical images may also be inferred from the brief personal details communicated about a person[49] (e.g. their age, marital status or occupation) and used to place the unknown person within a prototypical group. An individual's voice, style of dress or age can all influence how others perceive them. Stereotyping is the process of assigning people a category determined by one or a number of specific characteristics, and the allied assumption that they adopt other characteristics of that group, with all members of the group deemed to exhibit the same characteristics. For example, the stereotypical image of a 'granny' is of an apple-cheeked, kindly older woman with a predilection for baking apple pies, and such an image will have stereotypical expectations of behaviour associated with it.[49]

Hepworth[50] asserts the significance of an individual's appearance in people's perception of their age. He argues that we live in an increasingly 'visual culture' (p. 6), with vision often acting as the definitive sense. People interpret visual cues and decide whether people look old or young or somewhere in between. He described this physiognomic perception as an 'image of ageing' (p. 7), no more real or definitive than any other artefacts such as paintings, television programmes or sculptures. There are widely diverse ways in which images can be interpreted, or indeed manipulated, but these may be prejudiced by what might represent society's desire for images of 'artistic perfection' (p. 9).

The presence of stigma (unusual physical characteristics such as a physical disability or scarring) may suggest an abnormality or lack of ability in other respects.[49] Hepworth[50] describes the distaste expressed by individuals when viewing images of naked older people. These bodies were considered in quite derogatory and negative terms, possibly because they confront the individual with the realities of ageing, reinforced by connotations of both physical and mental decay. However, people can assume the appearance and outlook on life usually associated with someone several decades older.[51]

There is also a need for nurses to be aware that the way in which they regard their patient may shape and influence their judgement of them. Industrial and organisational psychologists have provided some insight into the ways in which 'first impressions' really do count. 'First impression error' occurs when the first judgement made by one individual about another will shape all subsequent judgements.[52] For example, if a nurse's first encounter with a patient involves preventing them from punching another patient who is usually quiet and passive, it is possible that they will make a sustained judgement that the first patient is a violent troublemaker.

Also to be considered is what has been termed the 'halo effect',[52] also known as 'halo error'. This occurs when the rater (nurse) judges on the basis of an overall impression. In other words, there is no differentiation between aspects of the patient that are actually quite different, such as cognitive function and mobility.[53] This may be because one particular characteristic is so striking that it obliterates other less distinct traits. Dipboye et al.[45] suggest that this would result in an overall rating of the individual on the basis of that one characteristic. They used the example of a student evaluating their lecturer. If the student considered the lecturer to be unenthusiastic about teaching, this might result in a negative evaluation of their teaching skills and subject knowledge. The converse would be true for a lecturer considered by their students to be enthusiastic.

Rater accuracy is also likely to be affected by the 'similar-to-me' effect. This means that the rater would be more sympathetic to individuals who share their outlook on life, or the same interests.[52] Other factors that have been found to influence raters' perceptions of an individual include physical attractiveness (unattractive people are more likely to receive lower ratings than more attractive people) and personal liking (raters are likely to rate people they like higher than those they do not like).[45]

Although the work of these theorists was focused on personnel management, it does allow some understanding of how the way in which a nurse regards the patient may influence the way in which he or she judges them. Nurses may be less motivated to regard patients sympathetically if they do not like them or find them otherwise unappealing. It can be seen that this may impair the objectivity of their judgements, and thus an assessment of that patient's needs.

Documentation and communication

A nurse may conduct assessments on both new and existing patients. If a nurse knows a patient, they will be able to draw on their own recollections of that patient, and will have an awareness of how that individual might behave in particular circumstances, their likes and dislikes, and how well they are able to communicate their needs. The nurse will have had the opportunity to get to know the patient's family and friends, and will have some views on how supportive and well informed they are. However, when assessing a new patient the nurse will have no prior knowledge of that person, and will be totally reliant upon the patient, their family and/or previous carers for information, while of course protecting the patient's right to confidentiality (*see* Chapter 7 for information relating to patient confidentiality).

Even when a nurse has been caring for a patient for some time, they will need to obtain information from other nurses and healthcare workers, because no nurse works 24 hours a day, seven days a week. Yet even when on duty the nurse will not be able to spend all their time with one patient. The effective communication of information is therefore vital if nurses are to be fully informed about their patient and able to make a reliable assessment.

Communication between nurses, patients and informal carers is explored in Chapter 6. The following section will consider communication between the nurse and other healthcare professionals.

Reasons for communication

It has already been acknowledged that older adults, particularly those entering long-term care, may have complex needs (*see* Chapter 2). In order to fulfil these needs it will be necessary to evaluate the patient's condition regularly, and to modify care as necessary. Communication will play a fundamental role in this, and may serve a number of purposes.[54] In the following examples, fictitious nurses describe how and why they communicate.

- *To make information available to other members of staff.* 'Mr Smith, well – he got quite snappy with me the other night, really abrupt and snatched his hand away. He wasn't his usual self at all, so I told them at handover and made sure I jotted it down in his notes as well.'
- *To obtain information from other members of staff.* 'I'd just come back from days off, and I wasn't sure what was happening with Fred's dressing. I was the only qualified nurse on duty, so there wasn't anyone else around to ask. I went and had a look at the notes and Jean, one of the other staff nurses, had written it all down. So that was OK.'
- *To monitor and evaluate the patient's progress.* 'Jim has had this sore on his leg for some time now – he came in with it. Each time we re-dress it we use a scale to evaluate it – size, depth, and so on. We make a record of this and this tells us that it is improving, slowly, but there is an improvement.'
- *To exchange ideas with other members of staff in order to make decisions more objective and reduce the effect of prejudicial (both positive and negative) attitudes to the patient.* 'I know that when it comes to Mary – well, I've got a bit of a soft spot for her. I find it hard sometimes to accept that she is going downhill, I don't want to see it, so it's good to have a chat with the other nurses about her. They sometimes see things that I don't (or don't want to!).'
- *To give instructions to/make requests of other members of staff.* 'If I am going to have a few days off I will make a note in the records for the other staff and ask them

to just check the dressing every day. It should be fine until I get back, but just to be sure . . .'

- *To fulfil legal and professional obligations.* 'We have to record when we have given medications, so that others will know that the patient has had them and do not administer them again.'
- *To provide legal protection – to 'cover ourselves'.* 'I would make a written record of the fact that they had got a little cut on their hand, just in case there was any kind of 'come back' from the relatives at a later date.'

Methods of communication

Communication between staff may be either verbal or written, and the way in which information is communicated verbally is likely to differ from that documented in a written patient record.[1] Verbal exchanges will be supported by hand gestures, facial expressions and alterations of voice tone, and these will enrich the information exchanged in ways that are not possible when making a written record. Of course, communication may be entirely non-verbal, but for the purpose of this section only written and verbal methods of communication will be considered.

Verbal communication may take place on an informal basis, for example in the corridor or at coffee break, with more formal verbal exchanges occurring on occasions such as staff handovers and ward rounds. However, in general it has been found that more information is recorded in the patient's notes than is exchanged verbally at handover,[1] with the added benefit of the former having a much wider potential audience than the latter. This indicates that written documentation may be the most effective means of communicating patient information. For example, Lamond found that verbal reports at shift handover were more likely to focus on what she termed 'global judgements'[1] – that is, information directly relating to the patient's current condition, the treatment and care that they are receiving, and factors relating to their personality and psychological state. Nurses generally communicated more information pertaining to the patient's psychological and social status in writing than they did verbally at handover.

This echoes the findings of Payne *et al.*,[55] who conducted research specifically into the handover interactions between nurses caring for older adults. Their study also indicates that nurses may rely heavily on jargon and abbreviations when communicating at handover, which some junior nurses may find difficult to understand. The handovers surveyed were often rushed and underplayed the nursing contribution to patient care, with the patient's resuscitation status being regarded as highly pertinent. Summary statements such as 'fine', 'OK' or 'poorly'[56] were used to describe the extent of nursing input to the patient's care, rather any detailed description of their nursing care needs. Team handovers were likely to focus on the nursing tasks that had already been completed and those that remained to be done by the subsequent shift, and verbal exchanges during the course of a shift were also likely to be goal directed. It was only during the informal discourse between the 'entering' and 'departing' shifts that any information relevant to the patient as a person was exchanged.

Requirements of communication

Nurses should comply with a number of requirements when communicating patient information. The first and perhaps most obvious one is to remember that if information is not communicated for any reason, it will not be available to others. I interviewed 28 nurses as part of my own investigation of the communication and acquisition of information practices of nurses caring for older patients.[54,56] I presented them with 48 cards describing various changes in physical/functional and psychological condition and asked them to select from a number of options stating:

1   where they were likely to go for additional information
2   how they were likely to communicate their observations.

For the majority of the scenarios, nurses stated that they would communicate the information to their colleagues in some way. Of these, in 65% ($n = 869$) of instances this would be in writing, and in 12% ($n = 165$) of cases nurses felt that communicating the information verbally would suffice. However, for 10% ($n = 134$) of the scenarios nurses stated that they would simply 'keep a mental note' of the information, and in less than 1% ($n = 17$) of cases the nurses felt that there was no need to communicate the information as it had no relevance to the patient's care needs. This information would not therefore be available to their colleagues.

Although most of the information that nurses said they would not communicate related to observations such as the patient opting not to participate in an activity that they had previously enjoyed, in other cases more serious scenarios were described. For example, four nurses (14%) stated that they would make only a mental note of their observations for the following scenario:

> Yesterday you gave the new patient (admitted shortly after you had
> been on a two-week leave) a bed bath. It passed without event. Today
> you do the same thing, but they make a loud and what you consider to
> be challenging sexual request of you.

One nurse explained that she would worry about the patient getting into trouble and being condemned by other staff if she communicated this information. Other nurses shared similar concerns. Although the nurses may respond differently when actually in practice, this finding does indicate that there may be instances when even very important pieces of patient information will not be communicated.

Why communication may not be effective

At this point it should be acknowledged that even when nurses do make a written record of their observations, this does not necessarily mean that information will be accessible to or actually used by other healthcare professionals. This may be for a number of reasons, which will each be considered in turn.

Nurses may make records that will only be accessed by themselves
Nurses may make a written record, but make it available to no one other than themselves, possibly in the form of aides-mémoire on pieces of paper kept in their uniform pockets, for example. These 'scraps' have been shown to be important 'hidden' sources of information.[57]

Although records make information available to a wide audience, other nurses may not actually access these records
The fact that information has been recorded does not mean that other members of staff will actually ever read it. Indeed, my research indicates that in some circumstances, nurses are more likely to consult the patient or other staff for information before 'going to the notes'.

Relevant observations may have been recorded by other members of staff, but not where the investigating nurse is looking[58,59]
Documentation is not a uniform process, and different institutions have different documentation practices. Even nurses working within the same institution or unit may have their own individual practices and motivations for making a particular documentary record. A total of 26 different documentation sites were mentioned by nurses participating in my research, and although different names may have been given for the same site (e.g. 'the patient's notes' may equate to 'nursing notes'), it does give some indication of the diversity of documentation sites (*see* Box 5.2). Information will effectively be 'lost' if a nurse does not know where to look for information, or looks for it in the wrong place.

Box 5.2 Documentation sites

Record of nursing care given/planned
1 Daily progress report
2 Progress notes
3 Daily notes
4 The patient's notes
5 Kardex
6 Daily record
7 Nurses' notes
8 Nursing notes
9 Care plan (new and existing)

Records of drug administration
10 Drug chart
11 Drug sheet
12 MARS sheet
13 Treatment/drug sheet

Records of specific assessment of patient status
14 Fluid balance chart
15 Tissue viability forms
16 Pressure sore forms
17 The patient's profile

Records made primarily by doctors
18   Doctors' notes
19   Medical notes

Nurse-made records of visits to the patient by other healthcare professionals
20   Special sheet for doctors' visits

Records giving specific information/instructions to colleagues
21   Communications page (entire multi-disciplinary team has access to this)
22   Communications book (record important information for the next shift to see)
23   Handover sheet
24   The diary

Records of patient care/status used by the multi-disciplinary team
25   The combined notes (for the use of both doctors and nurses)
26   Multi-disciplinary notes (for nurses, physiotherapists, etc.)

Other relevant observations have been recorded, but the record is not comprehensive enough to make the information available to the investigating nurse[60]

Nurses do not like documentation,[61] and they often resent the time that it takes. They may also underestimate the value of documentation, completing records only because of legal and/or professional requirements.[56] Furthermore, research indicates that even when records have been made, they often fail to adequately represent the nursing care given to a patient.[59,60,62,63] This is true even in cases where nurses feel that they have spent enough or too much time on their documentation. Nurses have also been found to significantly overestimate the quality of their written record.[60] Why might this be so? There are a number of reasons why documentation may fail to adequately represent patients and the care that they both need and have received.

1   Nurses may find it difficult to translate what they have seen, smelled or heard into prose.[64]
2   Nurses may lack the literacy skills necessary to make adequate written records. For example, nurses for whom English is not their first language or those with dyslexia may experience difficulties with written communication.[61]
3   A nurse's preferred style of writing may compromise their written expression of what they have observed.[65]
4   Institutions may require nurses to adopt a particular style of writing which conforms to professional and legal guidelines, but which may also serve to compromise the expression of what they have actually observed.[65]
5   Nurses may wish to avoid making a record of something that may leave them vulnerable either to criticism from their colleagues or to litigation. Nurses may also conceal facts by writing in such a way as to distance themselves from any possibility of 'blame', say, should the patient have an accident.[66] For example, if a patient is sometimes 'unsteady' and needs some supervision when mobilising, a nurse might be reluctant to record the fact that they were called away while escorting that patient to the toilet. To write the following

would not be a lie, but it would be a manipulation of the truth: *'Patient walked to the toilet with some supervision'*.

6   Nurses may forget to make a written record.

7   Nurses may for a variety of reasons choose not to make a written record.[55]

8   Nurses may make a written record in one part of the patient's records, but fail to transfer that information to other relevant areas.

Another nurse has made observations which they consider to be relevant to that patient's care, but have not documented them[59]

Despite the fact that there is evidence to suggest that time spent writing may not actually be 'excessive', nurses may resent the amount of time that they spend completing patient records, and feel that it impinges on the time that they can actually spend with patients.[67] This negative regard for the value of documentation[66] may diminish their motivation to make written records, and if a note is not made, then no written record of their observation will be available to other nurses, should they look for it.

Relevant observations have not been recognised as such by other nurses, and therefore have not been documented

Different people will interpret the same observation in different ways, and potential reasons for this have been explored in previous chapters. They include information-processing theory (*see* Chapter 4), the nurse's memory and recall of information, and the role of stereotypes and prejudicial images in the nurse's perception of the patient. A nurse may judge their observations on the basis of their previous experiences with that patient. They may evaluate as insignificant some observed behaviour which other nurses might regard as more worthy of note, and are therefore unlikely to document this observation. Furthermore, the nurse may simply lack the knowledge and experience necessary to recognise the significance of what they have observed (*see* Chapter 6).

Relevant behaviours have gone unnoticed by other nurses and therefore have not been documented

This may be for the reason cited in the previous paragraph, or the nurse may simply not have been with the patient at the relevant time (e.g. when they stumbled and almost fell in the corridor). As already stated, nurses cannot be with their patients 24 hours a day. If they are not there, they cannot see, and will be relying on the provision of information by others, including the patient, other healthcare workers or the patient's relatives. Chapter 6 explores reasons why the communication of this information may be unreliable.

Hostility between individuals or groups

There may be a lack of understanding between practitioners working in different clinical areas,[68] or even suspicion and hostility.[69] One nurse may dislike another, or regard a colleague as unapproachable. It is obvious that in circumstances such as these, unless a strong sense of professionalism prevails, both motivation to communicate and the efficacy of information transfer may be compromised. It is important to remember that we are communicating for the patient's benefit and not our own.

Although the factors outlined earlier in this chapter relate more specifically to written communication, they would also apply in principle to verbal communication.

It is clear that, regardless of the method of communication, it is important to ensure that the facts are accurate and made available to other personnel as appropriate, clearly and comprehensively, as soon as possible and without compromising patient confidentiality. Although many of these requirements are common sense, they are also enshrined in ethical, professional and legal guidelines, and breach of these may have potentially serious consequences for the quality of patient care, for the nurse and also for their employing organisation.

The Nursing and Midwifery Council[70] provides a very useful summary of guidelines for record keeping:.

- Record keeping is an integral part of nursing, midwifery and specialist community public health nursing practice.
- Good record keeping is a mark of the skilled and safe practitioner.
- Records should not include abbreviations, jargon, meaningless phrases, irrelevant speculation or offensive subjective statements.
- Records should be written in terms that the patient or client can easily understand.
- By auditing your records, you can assess the standard of the records and identify areas for improvement and staff development.
- You must ensure that any entry you make in a record can be easily identified.
- Patients and clients have the right of access to records held about them.
- Each practitioner's contribution to records should be seen as of equal importance.
- You have a duty to protect the confidentiality of the patient and client record.
- Patients and clients should own their healthcare records as far as is appropriate and as long as they are happy to do so.
- The principle of the confidentiality of information held about your patients and clients is just as important in relation to computer-held records as for all other records.
- The use of records in research should be approved by your local research ethics committee.
- You must use your professional judgement to decide what is relevant and what should be recorded.
- Records should be written clearly and in such a manner that the text cannot be erased.
- Records should be factual, consistent and accurate.
- You need to assume that any entries you make in a patient or client record will be scrutinised at some point.
- Good record keeping helps to protect the welfare of patients and clients.   (p. 14)

In summary

This chapter provides an overview of how nurses themselves may compromise the reliability of an assessment. The role of memory and the recall of information have been reviewed. It is clear that even if the nurse has once been in possession of information about a patient, they may not be able to remember it when it comes to making an assessment.

The possibility that a nurse's regard for their patients may be vulnerable to prejudice and bias is also considered. The way in which a nurse views their patient and the efficiency of their recall of pertinent information may significantly influence their assessment of an older patient.

This chapter concludes with an exploration of the role of documentation and communication in nursing practice. It outlines the importance of documentation as a way of communicating information. Although this is often resented as a tedious and time-consuming task, nurses should remember that what they write or neglect to write about a patient might have a profound effect on the care that the patient receives. The information that nurses communicate may also influence the practice of other professionals. Information that is not readily available in written format may not be available to the other healthcare professionals caring for the patient either at that time or at some stage in the future. It is not possible to communicate all information verbally. Even nurses who are caring for patients on a daily basis benefit from re-reading their own written records when monitoring patient progress. Inadequate documentation may not only reflect but also contribute to an ineffective assessment.

Key points

- Although there is some difficulty in defining an accurate decision, for the purpose of this book an accurate decision is one which appears to correlate with all of the other available evidence and which is not contradicted or challenged by other decisions or judgements made by the nurse.
- The accuracy of decisions and judgements may be compromised by factors such as impaired recall of observations, base rate neglect, the effect of the nurse's past experiences, hindsight bias, and stereotypical or prejudicial perceptions of the patient.
- If a nursing assessment of an older adult is to be accurate, then the judgements and decisions made as part of the assessment process will need to be accurate.
- If a nurse is to be fully informed about a patient and their needs/status, they will also need access to information obtained by other nurses and healthcare professionals.
- If such information is either not accessed or is communicated ineffectively, any relevant decision would be based on incomplete information, and its accuracy would be compromised.

References

1 Lamond D (2000) The information content of the nurse change of shift report: a comparative study. *J Adv Nurs.* **31:** 794–804.

2 Dowding D and Thompson C (2003) Measuring the quality of judgement and decision making in nursing. *J Adv Nurs.* **44:** 49–57.

3 Thompson C (1999) A conceptual treadmill: the need for 'middle ground' in clinical decision-making theory in nursing. *J Adv Nurs.* **30:** 1222–9.

4 Botti M and Reeve R (2002) Role of knowledge and ability in student nurses' clinical decision-making. *Nurs Health Sci.* **5:** 39–49.

5 Lamond D and Farnell S (1998) The treatment of pressure sores: a comparison of novice and expert nurses' knowledge, information use and decision accuracy. *J Adv Nurs.* **27:** 280–6.

6 Corcoran S (1986) Task complexity and nursing expertise as factors in decision making. *Nurs Res.* **35:** 107–12.

7 Benner P (1984) *From Novice to Expert: excellence and power in clinical nursing practice.* Addison-Wesley, Menlo Park, CA.

8 Harbison J (2001) Clinical decision-making in nursing: theoretical perspectives and their relevance to practice. *J Adv Nurs.* **35:** 126–33.

9 Cioffi J (2002) What are clinical judgements? In: C Thompson and D Dowding (eds) *Clinical Decision Making and Judgement in Nursing.* Churchill Livingstone, Edinburgh.

10 Crow RA, Chase J and Lamond D (1995) The cognitive component of nursing assessment: an analysis. *J Adv Nurs.* **22:** 206–12.

11 Dowding D (2002) Interpretation of risk and social judgement theory. In: C Thompson and D Dowding (eds) *Clinical Decision Making and Judgement in Nursing.* Churchill Livingstone, Edinburgh.

12 Royal College of Nursing (1997) *Royal College of Nursing Assessment Tool for Nursing Older People.* Royal College of Nursing, London.

13 Tanner CA *et al.* (1987) Diagnostic reasoning strategies of nurses and nursing students. *Nurs Res.* **36:** 358–63.

14 Lamond D, Crow R and Chase J (1996) Judgements and processes in care decisions in acute medical and surgical wards. *J Eval Clin Pract.* **2:** 211–16.

15 Lamond D *et al.* (1996) Information sources used in decision making: considerations for simulation development. *Int J Nurs Stud.* **33:** 47–57.

16 Taylor H. (2003) It's not what you do – it's the way that you do it. *Nursing Older People.* **14:** 32.

17 Australian National Institute of Clinical Studies (ANICS) (2003) *Information Finding and Assessment Methods that Different Groups of Clinicians Find Most Useful.* Prepared by the Centre for Clinical Effectiveness, ANICS, Melbourne.

18 Baddeley A (1996) *Your Memory: a user's guide.* Prion, London.

19 McGeoch JA and MacDonald WT (1931) Meaningful relation and retroactive inhibition. *Am J Psychol.* **43:** 579–88.

20 Brailey K, Vasterling JJ and Franks JJ (2001) Memory of psychodiagnostic information: bias and effects of expertise. *Am J Psychol.* **114:** 55–92.

21 Godden D and Baddeley A (1980) When does context influence recognition memory? *Br J Psychol.* **71:** 99–104.

22 Ericsson KA, Chase WG and Faloon S (1980) Acquisition of memory skill. *Science.* **208:** 1181–2.

23 Neath I (1998) *Human Memory: an introduction to research, data and theory.* Brooks/Cole Publishing Company, Pacific Grove, CA.

24 Paddock JR *et al.* (2000) When knowing becomes remembering: individual differences in susceptibility to suggestion. *J Genet Psychol.* **161:** 453–68.

25 Van Hook CW and Steele C (2002) Individual personality characteristics related to suggestibility. *Psychol Rep.* **91:** 1007–10.

26 Lane SM *et al.* (2001) How events are reviewed matters: effects of varied focus on eyewitness suggestibility. *Memory Cognition.* **29:** 940–7.

27 Rosenthal R (2002) Suggestibility, reliability, and the legal process. *Dev Rev.* **22:** 334–69.

28 Bain SA and Baxter JS (2000) Interrogative suggestibility: the role of interviewer behaviour. *Legal Criminol Psychol.* **5:** 123–33.

29 Trowbridge BC (2003) Suggestibility and confessions. *Am J Forens Psychol.* **21:** 5–23.

30 Thompson C (2003) Clinical experience as evidence in evidence-based practice. *J Adv Nurs.* **43:** 230–7.

31 Cioffi J (2001) A study of the use of past experiences in clinical decision making in emergency situations. *Int J Nurs Stud.* **38:** 591–9.

32 Cioffi J (1998) Decision making by emergency nurses in triage assessments. *Accid Emerg Nurs.* **6:** 184–91.

33 Tversky A and Kahneman D (1973) Availability: a heuristic for judging frequency and probability. *Cogn Psychol.* **5:** 207–32.

34 Tversky A and Kahneman D (1974) Judgement under uncertainty: heuristics and biases. *Science.* **185:** 1124–31.

35 Benner P, Tanner CA and Chesla CA (1996) *Expertise in Nursing Practice: caring, clinical judgement and ethics.* Springer Publishing Company, New York.

36 Benner P, Hooper-Kyriakidis P and Stannard D (1999) *Clinical Wisdom in Critical Care: a thinking in action approach.* WB Saunders Company, Philadelphia, PA.

37 Gardner H (1984) *The Mind's New Science: a history of the cognitive revolution.* Basic Books Inc., New York.

38 Thompson C (2002) Human error, bias, decision making and judgement in nursing – the need for a systematic approach. In: C Thompson and D Dowding (eds) *Clinical Decision Making and Judgement in Nursing.* Churchill Livingstone, Edinburgh.

39 Fischoff B (1982) Debiasing. In: D Kahneman, P Slovic and A Tversky (eds) *Judgement Under Uncertainty: heuristics and biases.* Cambridge University Press, New York.

40 Sanna LJ, Schwarz N and Stocker SL (2002) When debiasing backfires: accessible content and accessibility experiences in debiasing hindsight. *J Exp Psychol Learn Mem Cogn.* **28:** 497–502.

41 Hoffrage U, Hertwig R and Gigerenzer G (2000) Hindsight bias: a by-product of knowledge updating? *J Exp Psychol Learn Mem Cogn.* **26:** 566–81.

42 Roese NJ and Olson JM (1996) Counterfactuals, causal attributions, and the hindsight bias: a conceptual integration. *J Exp Soc Psychol.* **32:** 197–227.

43 Reece Jones P (1995) Hindsight bias in reflective practice: an empirical investigation. *J Adv Nurs.* **21:** 783–8.

44 Cioffi J (2000) Nurses' experiences of making decisions to call emergency assistance to their patients. *J Adv Nurs.* **32:** 108–14.

45 Dipboye RL, Smith CS and Howell WC (1994) *Understanding Industrial and Organizational Psychology: an integrated approach..* Harcourt Brace College Publishers, Fort Worth, TX.

46 Scrutton S (1990) Ageism: the foundation of age discrimination. In: E McEwen (ed.) *Age: the unrecognised discrimination.* Age Concern, London.

47 Coupland N and Coupland J (1995) Discourse, identity, and aging. In: JF Nussbaum and J Coupland (eds) *The Handbook of Communication and Aging Research.* Lawrence Erlbaum Associates, Inc., Mahwah, NJ.

48 Taylor HJ (2000) A caring moment with Margaret. In: A Ghaye and S Lillyman (eds) *Caring Moments: the discourse of reflective practice.* Quay Books, Dinton.

49 Hinton PR (1993) *The Psychology of Interpersonal Perception.* Routledge, London.

50 Hepworth M (1995) Images of old age. In: JF Nussbaum and J Coupland (eds) *The*

Handbook of Communication and Aging Research. Lawrence Erlbaum Associates, Inc., Mahwah, NJ.

51 Stuart-Hamilton I (2000) *The Psychology of Ageing: an introduction* (3e). Jessica Kingsley Publishers, London.

52 Szilagyi AD and Wallace MJ (1990) *Organisational Behavior and Performance* (5e). Scott, Foresman/Little, Brown Higher Education, Glenville, IL.

53 Saal FE and Knight PA (1988) *Industrial/Organisational Psychology: science and practice.* Brooks/Cole Publishing Company, Pacific Grove, CA.

54 Taylor H (2005) *The nursing assessment of older adults.* PhD thesis (unpublished), University College Worcester.

55 Payne S, Hardey M and Coleman P (2000) Interactions between nurses during handovers in elderly care. *J Adv Nurs.* 32: 277–85.

56 Taylor H (2004) *The sources and communication of information by nurses caring for older adults in 48 simulated clinical situations.* Fifth Annual International Research Conference, Transforming Healthcare Through Research, Education and Technology. 3–5 November, School of Nursing and Midwifery Studies, Trinity College Dublin.

57 Hardey M, Payne S and Coleman P (2000) 'Scraps': hidden nursing information and its influence on the delivery of care. *J Adv Nurs.* 32: 208–14.

58 Miller P and Pastorino C (1990) Daily nursing documentation can be quick and thorough! *Nurs Manag.* 21: 47–9.

59 Martin A, Hinds C and Felix M (1999) Documentation practices of nurses in long-term care. *J Adv Nurs.* 8: 345–52.

60 Idvall E and Ehrenberg A (2002) Nursing documentation of post-operative pain management. *J Clin Nurs.* 11: 734–42.

61 Taylor H (2003) An exploration of the factors that affect nurses' record keeping. *Br J Nurs.* 12: 751–8.

62 Abraham A (2003) Inadequate nursing care and the failure to keep adequate records. *Prof Nurse.* 18: 347–9.

63 Nordstrom G and Gardulf A (1996) Nursing documentation in patient records. *Scand J Caring Sci.* 10: 27–33.

64 Quirk R (1968) *The Use of English* (2e). Longmans, Green and Co. Ltd, London.

65 Gryfinski JJ and Lampe SS (1990) Implementing focus charting: process and critique. *Clin Nurse Specialist.* 4: 201–5.

66 Tapp RA (1990) Inhibitors and facilitators to documentation of nursing practice. *West J Nurs Res.* 12: 229–40.

67 Korst LM *et al.* (2003) Nursing documentation time during implementation of an electronic medical record. *J Nurs Admin.* 33: 24–30.

68 Robinson A and Street A (2004) Improving networks between acute care nurses and an aged care assessment team. *J Clin Nurs.* 13: 486–96.

69 Reed J and Morgan D (1999) Discharging older people from hospital to care homes: implication for nursing. *J Adv Nurs,* 29: 819–25.

70 Nursing and Midwifery Council (2005) *Guidelines for Records and Record Keeping.* Nursing and Midwifery Council, London.

Chapter 6

Sources of information in the assessment process

Sources of information: an overview

In Chapter 4 the relationship of judgements and decision making to the assessment process was established. In Chapter 5 it was also asserted that for nurses to make a judgement or decision, they must first either retrieve information stored in their memory, or obtain new information.

It has been said that for an assessment to accurately reflect the patient's abilities and health status, the information upon which it is based must be accurate. The concept of accuracy in decision making was defined in Chapter 5, which also explored information sources allied to the nurse making the decision and how the quality of this information will influence the reliability of the assessment.

Within nursing there has been a combined government and intraprofessional drive to promote research-based practice, or more recently the use of best evidence, as a basis for nursing practice.[1-5] However, Carnwell[1] voices some concern about the way in which the terms 'research-based practice' and 'evidence-based practice' are used without differentiation. She states that theorists have provided varying definitions of these terms. Subsequent to a review of the literature she concludes that a 'research project begins with identifying a problem to be investigated and ends with an outcome in the form of results and recommendations'. However, evidence-based practice 'will be defined as the systematic search for, and the appraisal of, best evidence in order to make clinical decisions that might require changes in current practice, while taking into account the individual needs of the patient'[1] (pp. 56–7). Therefore, although research findings may constitute part of the evidence being appraised, the two terms are not synonymous.

When writing this book I have endeavoured to substantiate any points or arguments that I make by relating them to the literature. I was educated within the era of 'research-based' nursing practice, and am firmly committed to basing practice on the best available evidence, as is the nursing profession in general. Indeed, many papers have been published which expound the beneficial effects of implementing research findings on practice in diverse nursing fields. For example, Halstead[6] explains how the nursing literature helped her to enhance the learning environment for student nurses on a day-surgery unit. Breen[7] was able to gain insight into how people with dementia learn through the use of published data. Other examples of the beneficial effects of putting research into practice include accounts by Freeman[8] and Lefler.[9]

When considering the actual and potential benefits of putting research findings into practice, and in view of the enormous commitment of time and other resources that is involved in conducting research, it might reasonably be expected that research findings and other forms of evidence should constitute the basis of any nurse's practice. However, this does not appear to be the case. The Australian National Institute of Clinical Studies (ANICS),[10] in its review of the evidence based healthcare information-finding and assessment literature, acknowledges that:

> Numerous resources and techniques are available to assist clinicians accessing evidence-based health care information. Individuals are likely to use different approaches in different situations. Similarly within a particular discipline individuals no doubt vary in the ways that they go about finding and accessing information to assist their clinical decision making. (p. 5)

ANICS[10] reviewed 32 papers investigating healthcare professionals' preference for information sources. In 50% of the studies the preferred source was found to be 'people', including 'self', 'other professionals' and 'the patient'. Other sources included books, journals, databases and education, and information from drug companies, advertisements and television programmes.

This review provides a useful insight into the diverse information sources utilised by healthcare professionals. However, an examination of where nurses actually obtain information as part of the decision-making process reiterates the heavy reliance on information obtained from oneself and other people, rather than from other sources (e.g. research or audits).

Indeed, research conducted by Thompson et al.[11] sought to investigate the sources of information that nurses cited as being most useful in guiding a specified clinical question. A case study was performed on a convenience sample of 108 nurses working on six surgical wards, six medical wards and three coronary care units in hospitals in northern England. The nurses were of various ages, and participated in a semi-structured interview. In addition, 56% of these nurses were also observed in practice by the researchers. The findings indicate that even within the culture of evidence-based nursing, the use of research-based evidence plays only a small role in informing the decisions of the sample nurses, who preferred instead to rely on 'human' information such as that received from nursing and other colleagues. This was perceived as more useful than the text and electronic research-based resources available to them.

There is a growing body of literature exploring the reasons for nurses not putting research into practice, or what has been variously termed the 'research practice gap'[12] and the 'theory practice gap'.[13,14] These reasons include restricted access to relevant literature in the clinical setting,[15] nurses dismissing theory as a result of confusion arising from a lack of agreement in the literature,[16] lack of efficacy of promotion of theory-based practice by some nurse educators,[13] a perceived drive towards positivist evidence at the expense of nurses' preferred sources of evidence (qualitative findings or personal knowledge),[4] a need to promote research awareness,[5] difficulties in translating knowledge obtained from empirical paradigms to nursing practice,[17] the need for nurses to develop their creative and generative thinking in conjunction with their critical thinking skills[18] and organisational barriers to implementing research-based practice.[19]

It is clear, therefore, that many decisions and judgements may not be based on the 'best evidence'. There may be sound and justified reasons for this. In the heat of a clinical crisis the opinion of a respected colleague may be both more accessible and more relevant than some lengthy and unreadable tome.

So where do nurses go for information?

It has already been said that nurses base their judgements and decisions on information from diverse sources.[20] Perhaps the first question should be 'Surely they should just ask the patient – the person being assessed?'. Unfortunately, this is either not done or is simply not possible. Possible reasons for this will be explored later. Nurses are therefore often reliant on information external to the patient. So how exactly are these information sources used by nurses in the process of assessing older adults in their care? The way in which this information may influence the quality of the assessment outcome will also be indicated. Some reasons for inconsistencies in the assessment process have already been cited in Chapter 4, and have been shown to involve the quality of information used and/ or the processing of that information.

The nurse making the assessment

Without both a depth of understanding and experience of caring for the older adult, nurses may not recognise and differentiate between the causes of behaviours that they observe in their patients (*see* Chapter 2). For example, an individual may be eating very little, and this could be for a number of reasons. They may be suffering from some gastrointestinal disease, anorexia nervosa, depression or a cognitive impairment that removes their recall of how to behave at mealtimes. The patient may have some problem with their peripheral vision so that they cannot actually see all of the food on their plate, or they may be affected by anosognosia. Conversely, they may simply be repulsed by the table manners of the person sitting next to them, or the food may not be to their taste.

Holden[21] describes a number of observable behaviours and suggests alternative neuropsychological explanations for them. For example, individuals may be unable to dress themselves. Neuropsychological reasons for this could include anosognosia, agnosia or dressing apraxia. Not only do nurses need to be aware of these possible explanations, but they should also be alert to other possibilities.

Nurses should also be aware that there might be a tendency to inappropriately dismiss changes such as loss of memory or physical dexterity in a way that would not occur in the case of a younger patient.[22] Conditions that, if detected, could be treated and rectified may be regarded as a 'natural' part of ageing and therefore something to be tolerated. For example, the symptoms of anaemia could be attributed to 'normal' age-related tiredness or decline in physical fitness.

The patient as a source of information

There has been a shift in the balance of responsibility in the provision of healthcare towards a more egalitarian state, supported both in nursing theory and in healthcare policy.[23] This necessitates the patient maintaining responsibility for their own health and their desire for autonomy and independence. This may not happen for a number of reasons (e.g. patient passivity[24]). Significantly, the contribution of the patient him- or herself as a tangible source of information in assessment is often ignored (e.g. what the patient has said, what the patient has told the nurse). Within a culture of patient-centred care it would reasonably be expected that the patient him- or herself would be the best source of this information.[25]

However, many of the studies of nurse decision making have been structured in such a way as to exclude 'what the patient tells me' as an actual or potential source of information. Why should this be? Some insight can be gained by looking at investigations into nurse decision making. These have made wide use of simulated clinical situations[26–28] (*see* Chapter 4), which preclude the patient's active contribution to the decision-making process.

It could be said that where studies have been based on simulated scenarios, the nurse would have no historical knowledge of the patient and how they react and respond in different situations. They will not know how they smell or sound. They will have no opportunity of knowing whether their tone of voice changes when they are experiencing discomfort, and the importance of this information will have been negated. This is significant in view of the findings of a study by Prescott *et al.*,[29] which indicate that the only factor to result in a significant difference in two nurses' ratings of a patient was the amount of prior knowledge the nurses had of that patient. This is not surprising, because 'without knowledge about the nature of people and their health-related needs, nurses would be unable to go about their work in anything but a haphazard way'[30] (p. 1). Yet the contribution of information obtained directly from the patient has been largely ignored in investigations into decision making.

Finding out what the patient wants

Effective assessment is vital if autonomy and independence for older people are to be promoted within the field of healthcare,[23] and if the person-centred care outlined in the *National Service Framework for Older People*[31] is to be achieved (*see* Chapter 2). However, this will be difficult if patients are not able or permitted to be actively involved in making decisions about their care[25] (*see* Chapter 2).

Although 'empowerment' is a term used frequently in nursing, with varying meanings, Rodwell's analysis[32] of the literature indicates that empowerment generally involves facilitating a client's autonomy. By working to develop their self-esteem and a sense of value, patients may be encouraged to take responsibility for their own health and for decisions concerning their life.[32] The nurse will need to accept that the client's decisions may have negative effects on their health, with a requirement for balance between minimising risk and promoting independence[23] (also *see* Chapter 7). Rodwell[32] indicates that for a nurse to be able to facilitate empowerment, they need to respect both their self and their practice. Without this, they would lack confidence in their judgements and decisions. Davies *et al.*[23] state that although independence is a term that is often used synonymously with autonomy in the literature, it might be viewed more appropriately as a factor necessary for the attainment of autonomy.

There is a dichotomy between the need to promote an individual's right to choice, autonomy and privacy[33] and the need to ensure that an individual has access to the services that they may require, the achievement of a balance being difficult. Caldock[34] surveyed social care workers following the last major reforms in assessment and delivery of care to older adults subsequent to the publication of *Caring for People*.[35] The sample of 40 individuals was selected to represent a range of social care workers working within two Welsh counties. Respondents participated in 33 interviews, some of which were group interviews. They expressed a concern that although the implementation of holistic assessments may reveal care needs that might otherwise have remained hidden, it is possible that these would conflict with older people's desires to maintain privacy, dignity and independence. There was a suspicion that the assessment and consequent delivery of care might be unresponsive to the wishes of individuals – an 'all or nothing' effect. The fear of this could, in reality, deter some older people from seeking assistance, or encourage them to conceal a need for assistance.

Consider the following scenario.

Jean is a community nurse with many years' experience. For several months now she has been visiting the home of Fred and Vera Atkins. Fred suffers from an Alzheimer's-type dementia, and his wife Vera is his main carer. Fred also suffers from diabetes. Generally, his condition has been deteriorating, and he is becoming more and more dependent on Vera. Jean has been visiting to treat an ulcer on Fred's left leg. Vera has always appeared to enjoy Jean's visits, and the two women often have an animated conversation putting the world to rights. During her most recent visit Jean realises that Vera is not her usual self. She also notices that the house looks untidy, and that Fred has not been shaved. Jean asks Vera if there is anything wrong. Vera becomes very defensive, and denies that there is a problem.

There could be a number of explanations for this situation.

1 Jean's visit was earlier than usual, and Vera had not had time to tidy the house and get both herself and Fred washed and dressed before Jean arrived.
2 Jean's visit was at the same time as usual, but Vera had not had time to tidy the house and get both herself and Fred washed and dressed before Jean arrived.
3 Jean's visit was at the same time as usual, but Vera had not been able to tidy the house and get both herself and Fred washed and dressed before Jean arrived.

But why did Vera become defensive? This might indicate that the third explanation was the most likely one. Why did she not explain this to Jean? Perhaps this was the reason.

I have always looked forward to Jean's visits. We have a good old chinwag, and some days when Fred is bad she is the only person I see all day that I can really have a chat *with*. I don't ever like her to think I am complaining, because I am not. 'For better or worse . . .' and all that, but some days it gets really hard. I am not getting any younger myself, and on the days when

> Fred's got it on him . . . well, I just feel like curling up in a ball and crying. But I can't, and I don't. That is not me. He is my husband and I love him. Sometimes when he lashes out. . . . Well, maybe then I don't like him too much. But it is not his fault, he doesn't know. I don't think he does anyway. He'll look at me, and it'll still be the Fred of old, and I know then – like I always know – that I will never let him go. I saw it in Jean's face today – that pity, that worry, 'the poor old dear can't cope'. Well, I can, and even if I couldn't I would never say. He is my husband, and he belongs here with me. So you will never get me to tell you anything that might make you take him away.

Perhaps you can now see why Jean appeared defensive.

How expectations of health service provision may influence older adults' use of services

Backett and Davison[36] suggest that expectations of health and health behaviours may be shaped by an individual's perception of what is reasonable or appropriate, and that this in turn will determine whether or not they seek healthcare. For example, younger adults with dependent children may be less tolerant of ill health and more willing to adopt a 'healthier' lifestyle than their elders.[36] These researchers suggest that older adults tend to base their ideas about health and illness on their own experiences of it, and are often dismissive of 'modern health fads', preferring to adopt a more common-sense approach to the manifestations of a lifetime of 'bad habits'. They are more likely to adopt an approach that accommodates rather than overcomes the status quo. Although younger adults generally have a sense that good health is a reasonably attainable objective, their older compatriots have a more realistic approach and make lifestyle choices that they consider to be reasonable, and have a more fatalistic attitude.[36] For example, an individual in their late eighties might consider it reasonable to eat and drink what they prefer, rather than adhering rigidly to a healthy eating plan. They would consider that any possible benefits of a low-fat diet would be outweighed by the pleasure of eating what their mood dictates. However, it must be made clear at this point that there are undoubtedly many older adults who fastidiously exercise and are careful about what they eat.

When making an assessment, the nurse will need to understand what aspects of the patient's health status are of concern to him or her, shaped by what it is possible and realistic to change or modify. Nurses also need to acknowledge that their own expectations for the patient's health may differ from those of the patient. There is potential for the nurse's expectations to fall anywhere between two extremes of a continuum. At one extreme would be the belief that if the older adult makes certain changes to their lifestyle all their health problems will be overcome. At the other extreme would be the expectation that because of the patient's advanced age and general state of degeneration, no positive changes to their state of health may be expected. Nurses should exercise caution and ensure that they do not impose their own health values when assessing the needs of their older patients. Being able to walk only as far as the kitchen and back might sound restrictive, but it could mean the difference between maintaining independence at home and being admitted to a care home.

Older adults, like younger ones, will have their own individual preferences for health outcomes,[37] and there is some debate in the literature as to whether older adults are more likely to opt for quantity rather than quality of life, or vice versa. Some individuals who are suffering from considerable ill health may wish to live as long as possible regardless of their state of health, while others would willingly exchange increased length of life for an improved health status for their remaining time. Furthermore, research has indicated that, given the choice, some older adults might wish for their life to end if they were resident in a nursing home in a confusional state, and to a lesser extent if they were suffering from functional limitations or pain.[38] However, these were responses to hypothetical rather than real situations, and someone may react very differently when confronted with the situation in real life. Indeed, in a study by Sherbourne *et al.*[37] it was found that 71% of adults aged over 80 years would be unwilling to forego any of their life in exchange for excellent health (compared with 93% of those aged 18–24 years). However, these respondents were self-reporting to be in good or excellent health. Those older respondents in the study who were willing to exchange some months of their life for perfect mental and physical health were more likely to be in less than perfect health than their younger counterparts.

Although the findings of neither of these studies[37,38] can be generalised to the older population as a whole, they do highlight the diversity of older people's expectations and preferences. Whilst nurses may have their own opinions about their patients' quality of life, they should understand and respect the fact that the opinions of their older patients may differ significantly from their own, and also that the opinions of these patients may vary over time. What an individual who is enjoying good health may deem to be an unacceptably low quality of life may become more tolerable and acceptable as their health status deteriorates. The literature indicates that nurses should exercise caution if they are to ensure that they do not impose their own health values when assessing the needs of their older patients.

When patients are unwilling or unable to make a reliable contribution to the assessment process

Stuart-Hamilton[39] describes confabulation as the 'making up of stories or implausible explanations to cover up gaps in memory or other skills' (p. 177). To the unaware observer, it is not uncommon to be deluded in this manner by someone with cognitive impairment. During new encounters it can be difficult to recognise that someone is disorientated or confused. Patients with even a moderate cognitive impairment (e.g. those with progressive dementias) may confabulate. The patient may provide convincing accounts of how they are able to maintain their activities of living independently, recounting trips to the shops and spring-cleaning sprees when in reality they are unable to perform these tasks.

It has already been suggested that patients may be unwilling to participate in the care process (*see* Chapter 2) either because they have an expectancy of dependency, or because they reject either consciously or subconsciously the concepts of independence and autonomy. Baltes[24] conducted research into different types of learned or imposed psychosocial dependency, an awareness of which may provide insight into an individual's behaviour. In their assessment, the nurse should therefore be aware of and differentiate between the different origins of dependency, described by Baltes as follows.[24]

- *Learned helplessness*: An individual suffers an injury or illness and in the early phases of their recovery they experience pain or discomfort when attempting to rehabilitate. Their efforts are not positively recognised by those caring for them, so they lose confidence in their own ability to recover and are thus discouraged from doing so.
- *Learned dependency*: In the early phases of recovery from an illness or injury, despite their recovering ability to self-care, an individual's carers are unwilling to allow them to do so. Even though a full or partial recovery of independence is physically possible, the individual allows their needs to be fulfilled by others.
- *Selective optimisation with compensation*: The individual recognises that it will not be possible for them to regain their pre-incident functional ability. They decide which aspects of function are important to them, and strive to regain these at the expense of independence in others.[24]

> Dependency due to old age is in part the outcome of society's negative attitude towards old age. It is more a self-fulfilling prophecy than a reflection of the true competence level of the elderly. (p. 1)

If patients are to be provided with appropriate care, there is a need to establish the reasons why they may not be able to perform specific functions. For example, it would be necessary to differentiate between an inability to dress oneself because of some physical explanation, such as restricted mobility following a cerebral infarct,[21] and an inability arising from dependency, including that imposed by organisational structures within society.[24] It is clear that occupational therapy and physiotherapy would be of greater benefit in the former case than in the latter.

An example of dependency imposed by organisational structures would be when an individual requests help for something with which they have been experiencing difficulty, but societal structures will not permit them to receive assistance only with this need, because of the inclusive nature of care packages. For example, Mrs Smith might have been experiencing difficulty getting in and out of the bath. Home care services were arranged not only to help her in and out of the bath, but also to help her to dry herself and get dressed after her bath. A nurse making an assessment based on records of the care package being delivered might reasonably conclude that Mrs Smith was unable to dry and dress herself – as indeed she may not by this stage, as she may have adopted a behavioural dependency.[24]

The danger is that both nurses and their patients may perceive dependency as being a permanent and inevitable part of ageing – an ageist perception[40] (*see* Chapter 5). However, Baltes[24] contests this view and asserts that with support and encouragement individuals can resume the ability to perform functions, if they are willing to embrace the concept of independence. Sometimes, however, people may prolong a dependent state out of fear of losing all forms of assistance, or the company of the care worker who has been assisting them.[41]

It could be concluded that recognition, and interpretation of, and differentiating between dependent behaviours are likely to be difficult when based upon subjective observations and reports from the patient and their caregivers. It may not be possible to determine which behaviours result directly from the physical manifestations of an illness or disease, and which have been learned.

The effects of patient expectations of nursing care

The delivery of healthcare may have changed quite considerably during the lifetime of older patients. Webster[42] describes how, at the outbreak of the Second World War, more than 60 000 chronically or acutely sick or simply infirm elderly were resident in public assistance institutions, which were still thought of as 'workhouses'. This was despite the 1929 Local Government Act, which stipulated that these people should be cared for in hospitals. These buildings were usually old and run down. Inspections made in preparation for the introduction of the NHS condemned 84% of the beds in South Wales as being 'unfit for improvement'.[42]

As a student nurse in the late 1980s I can still recall patients on the elderly care wards becoming distressed about being admitted to 'the workhouse'. These wards were based in what had indeed once been the workhouse, and many of the patients still saw it as such. Admission was something to be avoided, and this may well have influenced how they accommodated their health problems. To an extent this attitude arguably persists today in the older old.

Webster[42] provides an image of a post Second World War elderly working-class population who had borne the brunt of poor medical and welfare care. Women suffered the effects of inadequate maternity care, and few had their own teeth. There was an expectation of discomfort and incapacity. An awareness of the inadequacies of healthcare services before the introduction of the NHS and the modern welfare state could explain why older adults were reportedly more satisfied with NHS services than were younger people[31] – they simply have lower expectations. Indeed, Simmons and Schnelle[43] reported that the very elderly, frail, female and dependent residents of nursing homes were likely to have lower expectations of their carers than their younger, male and less dependent counterparts. It could reasonably be assumed that if patients have low expectations of healthcare, then they will make low voluntary demands of healthcare providers.

Yet again, however, there is evidence which suggests the need to exercise some caution and be aware that individuals will have their own personal beliefs and preferences, which shape the care that they expect to receive.[44] Research on the psychosocial preferences of a group of older adults found that the group greatly valued privacy, the right to self-determination, the freedom to control and choose their own social interactions, and the opportunity to participate in fulfilling and enriching activities. Although this study has limitations in that its sample group of 20 subjects (11 men and nine women), whilst all aged over 60 years, could not be considered representative of the general population of adults of this age (all of them were in reasonable health and were highly educated gerontologists), it does highlight the importance of nurses considering what is important for their patients when making an assessment: 'Providing individualised care depends, however, on the availability of comprehensive, reliable and valid ways of assessing what is important to individuals'[44] (p. 346).

A study by Bowers et al.[45] investigated how residents in three long-term care institutions rated quality of care, and indicates that a patient's sense of what is important is related to their level of dependency. Those with lower dependency levels tended to relate the quality of care to the service that they received. The 'care-as-service' group was often frustrated by what they considered to be the inattentiveness and lack of responsiveness of carers to their service needs. The prompt serving of food and drinks was considered important by this group, who were often labelled as 'complainers' by staff. However, the majority of respondents in this study referred to the service aspects of care only when prompted, valuing the interpersonal interaction with their carers more highly. This was termed the 'care-as-relating' group. Carers who were kindly and supportive and considered the patient as something more than a helpless dependent were excused omissions in other more physical aspects of care. This group did not consider having to wait as being indicative of poor care, and often made excuses for their carers. They frequently attempted to ease the burden on their carers by restricting their calls for help.

In a third group of more frail and dependent residents, great value was attached to care staff satisfying the resident's comfort needs – this was the 'care-as-comfort' group. These individuals often had an impaired ability to read and interpret body cues (e.g. the need to go to the toilet). They became wary about asking repeatedly for the same help in case they had misread cues. They sensed that the staff were irritated when taking them to the toilet for what often proved to be a false alarm. This group tended to wait until they became unbearably uncomfortable before asking for help, rather than incur the wrath of care staff. The fulfilment of these comfort needs was considered much more important than other aspects of personal or nursing care. However, whilst these findings are interesting, the method of sampling may prove limiting. The 26 participants were recruited from three long-term care institutions in the USA. Nurses selected the sample and excluded those individuals whom they regarded as either too ill or too cognitively impaired to participate in an in-depth interview. It could be said that this would render the sample unrepresentative of the general nursing home population.

There may be discrepancies in nurse and patient assessment of need.[46] There may also be conflict between nurses' perceptions of what is important for their older patients, and what the patients themselves consider to be important.[47] Indeed, Pearson et al.[48] collected data from a convenience sample of 1374 Australian nurses and nursing home residents over a two-year period and found that although there was a relatively high reported level of resident satisfaction with care in nursing homes, this did not always correlate with observer perceptions of quality of care and quality of life. This could mean either that observers' perceptions of quality of care were flawed or based on different criteria to those of the residents, or that the residents may have been reluctant to criticise staff.

Nurses need to be aware that now, in the 21st century, people's expectations of the NHS and thus the provision of healthcare in general may be very different from expectations during the first half of the last century.[42] Older people grew up in an era when there was a relative lack of availability of state-provided healthcare, and privately funded healthcare was too expensive for them to use.

The seeking of healthcare from a qualified professional was often simply not an option. Even though the situation has changed, the literature indicates (*see* Chapters 1 and 2) that older patients may still be unwilling to ask for assistance, or may simply not be aware that help is available. They may also remain uncomplaining when receiving poor-quality or inadequate care. This may be difficult for younger nurses to understand and acknowledge when caring for older people, but it is essential that such awareness exists.

The effects of culture and taboos

Nurses need to be aware that there will be times when their patients will not wish to disclose information to them because to do so may cause them embarrassment. There may also be situations when patients regard certain topics as taboo, and will therefore be unwilling to discuss them with the nurse. Such awareness will help the nurse to recognise the difficulties that their patient may be experiencing, and will enable them to make provision for the privacy and time that may be necessary if the patient is to be encouraged to be open with their nurse.

When the patient is embarrassed

In an era when matters of intimate physical functioning (e.g. menstruation) are freely discussed socially and in the media, it should be remembered that this has not always been the case. For example, the advertising of sanitary products on television has only been permitted since 1989, and then only after the 9pm 'watershed'.[49] A family medical reference book published in the 1920s[50] provides a useful insight into the attitudes of at least the upper middle classes of the day to a variety of health-related issues. In the chapter dedicated to 'female diseases', the authors state:

> Involving considerations of a delicate nature, these complaints have too generally and too long been shut out from works intended for popular distribution. Hence there is a general ignorance of a class of diseases . . . and the subjects of these maladies are generally themselves so uninformed of the true nature of their sufferings, that they are neither prepared to seek relief in the proper direction, nor to submit to the remedy if it chance to be proposed. (p. 415)

Such ignorance and sense of 'delicacy' may be difficult for young people in the 21st century to comprehend. It is useful for healthcare professionals today to gain insight into what it was permissible to discuss or even publish in the first quarter of the 20th century.

Patients may experience embarrassment if they are receiving care from a nurse of the opposite sex, and this may inhibit their communication with the nurse, as someone who is embarrassed or has something to hide may steer questions and thus attention away from the taboo subject. Although this is likely to affect patients of either sex, research does indicate that women are less willing to accept intimate care from male nurses than male patients are from female nurses, and that this situation has changed little over the past 20 years.[51]

When a subject is taboo

Assessment and expression of a subjective experience may be significantly influenced by ethnic and cultural factors.[52] In many cultures and societies any form of mental illness is still considered taboo. When assessing individuals from such groups, information concerning the taboo illness is less likely to be made available than that for other illnesses. Patients may also be reluctant to divulge information that they think will meet with the nurse's disapproval (e.g. self-inflicted suffering such as a hangover, or smoker's cough).

Different generations, cultures and societies will all have their own taboos, and nurses need to be aware that a patient's desire to avoid discussing these issues may influence the information that they give to the nurse.

Cognitive impairment

Assessment of the older adult is fraught with the difficulties associated with age-related mortality and pathology (*see* Chapter 2), and affected individuals may lack the ability to communicate information or understand what nurses are asking them.

Both cognitive impairment[53] and depression are notoriously poorly diagnosed and difficult to assess in older adults.[54–56] This is worrying in view of the fact that depression is considered to be one of the most prevalent mental health disorders among nursing home residents.[57]

There is even a lack of agreement on the definitive criteria for cognitive impairment, and this can result in differences in the evaluation of its incidence.[58] Researchers in this area have used a variety of different selection criteria for their studies, and not only is cognitive impairment assessed in different ways, but also terms such as 'dementia' and 'cognitive impairment' have been variously defined.[59–61] One definition of 'mild cognitive impairment', and that most commonly adopted in the literature, is 'a generic term for all cognitive changes observed in ageing'[58] (p. 403). It might therefore be concluded that as cognitive state declines it would be reclassified as first 'moderate' and then 'severe' accordingly.

Bischkopf *et al.*[58] also argue that 'cognitive impairment might fluctuate over time and is far too heterogeneous to define a specific circumscribed diagnostic category of high predictive validity' (p. 409), and they suggest that it is a state that may or may not develop into a pathological dementia. Differences in the definitions employed across studies will therefore mean that prevalence figures may differ. The Office for National Statistics[61] reports an incidence of cognitive impairment (and distinguishes this from dementia) of 16.6% of adults aged 60–64 years living in private households, rising to 25% in the group aged 70–74 years. The incidence of cognitive impairment increases with age, and this rise occurs at a younger age in women than in men. Cognitive impairment is also associated with increased care needs in other areas.

Tait and Fuller[59] have presented the findings of the *Health Survey for England 2000* report on the psychosocial well-being of older people. The sample consisted of adults aged 65 years or older living in private households or care homes. A total of 1677 individuals were interviewed at private addresses, and 2493 individuals were interviewed in care homes. Of the care home interviews, only 1220 interviews were conducted with the individual concerned, and 51% were conducted with a proxy. In total, 41% of the care home residents were considered by staff to be incapable of being interviewed in person. This was due to either a cognitive impairment or some other factor. In these cases a shortened interview was conducted with the proxy; this was also the procedure for those individuals who had a high score on the cognitive impairment scale. It was found that 19% of the nursing home residents and 22% of the residential home residents had some cognitive impairment. In total, 95% of those in private households and 49% of those in care homes were judged to have no impairment, with 2% and 33%, respectively, having a severe impairment.

Although these results are interesting, some caution should be exercised when interpreting them. Not only is cognitive impairment difficult to diagnose,[54–56] but the assessment process itself can actually cause confusion and anxiety, which could then present as impairment. This theory is supported by Chiriboga et al.,[53] who suggest that simply being aware that their cognitive ability is being tested could be enough to induce anxiety in patients, because the diagnosis of cognitive impairment is not a welcome or pleasant prospect. There is therefore a suggestion that the process of cognitive testing may in itself have a deleterious effect on the reliability of the test results. Furthermore, the anxiety associated with relocation to a nursing home may also contribute to an individual's sense of confusion. They will no longer be in familiar surroundings with people whom they know and love. Their meals may be served at different times, by people who are unaware of their preferences. Moving to a nursing home really is a significant and often traumatic experience, and it should be expected that it will have some impact on the patient's cognitive state. It might be suggested that it would be rather strange if it did not. Indeed, when Magaziner et al.[62] surveyed 2285 people aged over 65 years and newly admitted to a sample of 59 selected nursing homes in Maryland, USA, between 1992 and 1995, they found an incidence of dementia of around 50%. It is therefore possible that such a high prevalence of confusional state was associated with the enormous upheaval of nursing home admission, rather than with any pathological disorder.

Keady and Bender[63] have proposed that being assessed could put the individual concerned in a position of subordination and the assessor in a position of power. This can lead to a sense of loss of control, with the person being assessed worrying about the possible implications of the assessment outcome – a not unreasonable fear of being admitted to a care home and the loss of their freedom (the ethical implications of power relations in decision making are explored in Chapter 7). Furthermore, there is an argument that many of the tests for cognitive impairment are based on the assumption that the person being tested actually has some awareness of social context.[63] In view of the fact that not everyone does know who the Prime Minister is, and that it is easy to lose track of time and date when one is in a care home or other strange place, there is a belief that doctors may misdiagnose around 50% cases of dementia.[63]

In addition, there is some suggestion that the tests used for diagnosing cognitive impairment may not be culturally sensitive and may be unsuitable for translation into languages other than the one in which they were devised, or for use with one cultural group when they were designed for use with another.[64] This would have implications for those making an assessment of non-English-speaking individuals using an assessment tool designed for use with English speakers. One tool may not be suitable for use with all members of a culturally diverse community[64] (*see* p. 84 for further consideration of cognitive impairment).

Possible implications of being diagnosed as 'cognitively impaired'

Sansone *et al.*,[65] in their review of the literature, suggest that for healthcare professionals the diagnosis of dementia is usually perceived as being synonymous with the decline in judgemental ability or decision-making function. This may be associated with a professional desire to reduce 'risk', or the possibility of the patient making an 'unsafe' decision. This means that although the whole concept of decision-making capacity (i.e. how a person's competence to make decisions is determined) is ambiguous and open to interpretation, people with dementia are often deprived of the right to make choices and decisions.[65] This is despite research evidence from Sansone *et al.*[65] which indicates that a proportion of individuals with even severe cognitive impairment are able to make consistent healthcare choices over a three-week period, with the proportion rising considerably for those with only a mild impairment. Similarly, research conducted by Feinberg and Whitlatch[66] suggests that people with mild to moderate cognitive impairment are able to provide consistent responses when asked demographic questions about themselves, their preferences and their choices. Further support for the decision-making capability of people with dementia is provided by Moye *et al.*,[67] who investigated the ability of 88 volunteer older adults with mild to moderate dementia to give informed medical consent. They were compared with 88 matched controls using three instruments that measured understanding, appreciation, reasoning and ability to express a choice. It was found that although the test group exhibited some limitation to their understanding of treatment and information concerning the treatment, most of them were considered legally competent to make decisions. However, there were limitations to this study, including the selection criteria for the sample and the fact that the research tool had only recently been developed, and its validity and reliability were still being investigated.

Although it is important to acknowledge that individuals with a cognitive impairment may be able to make decisions and choices, nurses may not always be able to correctly identify which of their patients are able to do so. An investigation by Simmons and Schnelle[68] casts doubt on nurses' ability to identify those residents who are able to accurately report on their own health status and the care interventions that they receive. Variations in the condition of the patients and fluctuations in their confusional state may also contribute to difficulties in identifying those individuals with cognitive impairment who are able to consistently state a choice.[65]

Some caution should be exercised when considering the findings of studies involving patients with cognitive impairment, as the selection criteria may be flawed. For example, in a study by Pearson *et al.*[69] investigating resident satisfaction with quality of care in nursing homes, those residents who were unable to respond because of their cognitive state were excluded from the study. The researchers state[69] that some residents who were randomly selected for interview had been excluded because of their cognitive state. They acknowledge that this was unfortunate, but state that alternative ways of involving these subjects in the research (e.g. using advocates) would take too much time, and that there was a lack of literature to support this method.

Sensory impairment

The senses are the data sources of the brain and thus its means of contact with internal and external environments. Any decline in sensory acuity will not only impair the input of data (and therefore the quantity and quality of the information that the brain can access), but will also compromise intellectual functioning.[39] Such a decline is often associated with ageing. For example, older adults may need to be exposed to visual stimuli for longer than younger adults if their brain is to be able to identify the object that is being seen.[39] Visual recognition may therefore be impaired, and the processing of visual stimuli is also slower. Facets of hearing may also be defective.[39]

An understanding of how, for some people, sensory acuity may decline with age is important for nurses who are caring for older adults. This is because an impaired sensory input may have significant effects both on the way that an individual interprets their environment, and on the way that they react to stimuli. This may have a resulting effect on both their behaviour and their coping responses.[70] For example, hearing loss is known to make social interactions difficult and can lead to social isolation and depression. There is also evidence of an association between hearing loss and physical functioning.[71]

Individuals with a sensory impairment are likely to have developed compensatory mechanisms by which they can overcome their difficulties and live their daily lives,[70] and these are very important.[72] For example, they may use their sense of touch and feel their way along walls, rather than see when they have reached the foot of the stairs. A light may be connected to the doorbell so that a deaf person can see, rather than hear, when someone is at the front door. Such accommodatory facilities may not be available outside the home, and unless such sensory impairment is accommodated in another way, the ability of the individual to maintain their functional status may be compromised. Illness or other changes in health status may also mean that they are no longer able to maintain their compensatory mechanisms.

On a practical level, sensory impairment can also impinge on communication between the nurse and the patient.[73] Both nurses and patients can become frustrated by thwarted attempts to communicate, and nurses working in pressurised conditions may lack the time or patience to effect communication. Patients may feel reluctant to attempt to communicate their needs,[73] especially if nurses are unwilling to adopt established alternative methods of communication.

How many nurses, at the end of a busy shift, have rushed up to a patient with a hearing impairment, dashed off a series of questions and then scurried off to document that the patient was 'comfortable and had made no complaints'? Of course they hadn't – they had not been given the opportunity to do so. In the same vein, even where nurses are sensitive to a patient's hearing impairment, how willing would a patient be to discuss some intimate problem knowing that the nurse would be likely to bellow, for all to hear, *'So you have got some problems down below . . .'*? (For information relating to a patient's right to privacy, *see* Chapter 7.)

Maintaining the grasp of a conversation can be very tiring for a hearing-impaired person, and they may give up if the person to whom they are listening fails to accommodate this difficulty.[74] When 'listening' to a lip-read conversation, the hearing-impaired person has to amalgamate information from a number of sources, both visual and (to varying extents) auditory. There is room for error and misunderstanding in this interpretation.[74] If the nurse is aware of and sympathetic to this difficulty they will allow the patient time to think about what he or she is 'hearing' and provide the facility for feedback and correction. If not, then the communication between nurse and patient will be impaired. Nurses should also be aware that people with hearing loss are very sensitive to body language. If they sense that the nurse is becoming irritated at their lack of grasp of the conversation, they may withdraw from the conversation, with an adverse effect on the assessment process.[73]

Pain measurement

Difficulties associated with the general process of assessment were examined in Chapter 2. Nurses will also need to consider the difficulties that are encountered when assessing specific areas of patient need, and the assessment of pain in the older adult will be explored as an example of this. Older people are more likely to experience pain than their younger counterparts due to the combined effects of general physical degeneration and increased susceptibility to disease, and as a result of these factors their psychological, physiological and behavioural responses to pain may be altered.[75]

People cope with and express their pain in different ways, and the way in which a physical pain is experienced will be influenced by past experiences.[75,76] Each individual's experience and each episode of pain will therefore differ. Helman[77] suggests that whether the individual perceives the pain to be 'normal' or 'abnormal' may influence their communication of it, as will societal norms. If pain is considered within the context of suffering, then how the pain is borne will be influenced by societal and cultural expectations. For example, if the pain is the result of a behavioural transgression (e.g. a headache resulting from overindulgence in alcohol), then it is more likely to be suffered without fuss than if it was sustained in an unwarranted physical attack.

Pain is a highly individual and subjective experience, and the assessment of pain may therefore be vulnerable to the nurse's prejudice, with nurses possibly believing that older people have reduced sensibility to pain.[78] Hayes[79] suggests that even when nurses observe pain-related behaviours in older adults, they are likely to dismiss their observations or believe that the patient was imagining the pain. Age-related changes might make the expression of pain difficult, and unresolved pain can result in behaviour changes, loss of appetite, insomnia and impaired mobility.[79] These may have a concurrent effect on the patient's general health status and exacerbate the pain.

A study conducted by Ferrell et al.[80] found that in a sample of 97 institutionalised elderly patients, only 15% of the 75% of patients who were suffering pain had received analgesia during the last 24 hours. One can surmise that pain remains unresolved because of a combination of factors, including nurses not detecting pain, nurses not responding to observations of pain, patients not anticipating a helpful response from nurses so not reporting pain, and patients being unable to report episodes of pain.

The reporting of pain may also depend on the patient's expectations of helpful interventions from a nurse. Indeed, in an audit conducted by Simons and Malabar,[81] 10% of the patients in an elderly care unit who had said that pain was a problem had not told a nurse about their pain, simply because it was chronic pain and they did not think that the nurse would be able to help. The sample was recruited from patients admitted to three hospital wards (acute, rehabilitation and combined rehabilitation/continuing care). However, only patients whom the researchers had deemed able to communicate were eligible for inclusion, which meant that of a total of 140 new patients, only 105 patients were included in the study. The communication of pain was therefore not investigated for a large group of patients who, it could be argued, reflect some of the special needs associated with older adulthood.

There is an indication that even when pain is detected and measured by nurses, this information may not always be communicated to or made available to other nurses (*see* Chapter 5). Although nurses may record in writing that a patient has experienced pain, these records are unlikely to communicate effectively the nature of the pain.[82] Camp compared patients' descriptions of pain with nurses' documentation of pain assessments.[82] The convenience sample consisted of 84 nurse–patient dyads recruited in an American teaching hospital. The findings indicate that the sample nurses documented considerably less than 50% of the pain reported by their patients, with records focusing specifically on the pain locus, medication administered and the fact that the patient had complained of pain.

A patient's expressions of pain may also be subject to misinterpretation. Simons and Malabar[81] found that when a nurse interpreted behaviour as an expression of distress in patients with communication problems and/or cognitive impairment, they were more likely to think that the patient was hungry or thirsty rather than experiencing pain. However, when pain behaviours were observed, in the majority of cases interventions by nurses helped to modify these to non-pain behaviours. There are, however, limitations to this study. The researchers did not define what they considered to be 'communication problems' or 'confusional state'. They also failed to specify what they had defined as pain and non-pain behaviours, indicating that the research was based on the subjective opinions of individual nurses conducting the research, and different people may interpret behaviours in different ways. A number of behaviours have been associated with pain, including 'grimacing/frowning', 'restlessness', 'guarding or rubbing the painful part' and 'aggressive behaviour'[83] (p. 28). Zwakhalen *et al.*[84] conducted a cross-sectional study of a sample of Dutch nurses working with patients with severe intellectual disability. A total of 109 nurses (response rate of 81%) completed and returned a questionnaire rating 158 expressions of non-verbal pain behaviour on a 10-point scale. Although the researchers urge some caution (because of the large number of questions compared with the relatively small sample), the findings indicate that all 158 non-verbal descriptors such as moaning or crying while being handled, and facial expressions of pain, were regarded as being important indicators of pain. However, any of these descriptors could be manifestations of a number of other factors and entirely unrelated to pain. Conversely, the absence of any of these indicators does not necessarily mean that the patient is not experiencing pain, especially if they have suffered a cerebrovascular accident or they have Parkinson's disease, for example.[81]

Concerns were voiced by Fries *et al.*[85] that cognitive impairment is often associated with a decline in the reporting of pain, despite the fact that individuals with cognitive impairment may well have a lower general health status than those without such impairment. In the discussion of their validation of the Minimum Data Set Pain Scale, they infer that the recognition of pain severity in individuals with communication and/or cognitive impairment might be dependent upon the subjective interpretation of observers.

Hayes[79] also questions the quality of pain assessments in older people who are confused and/or unable to communicate verbally. Research by Wynne *et al.*[86] indicates that many pain assessment instruments, including the visual analogue scale, verbal rating scales and the Wong-Baker Faces Scale, are inappropriate for the assessment of pain in cognitively impaired nursing home residents. They found that for a group of patients with a Mini-Mental State Examination (MMSE) score of less than 15, describing the pain verbally and pointing to the pain were the most useful methods of indicating pain levels. Hayes[79] suggests that patients suffering from confusion might experience difficulties with understanding and following instructions on how to use a scale and then translating their perception of pain on to a visual scale. Hayes[79] also argues that chronic pain with an insidious onset might be more difficult to describe than acute pain.

A literature review by Briggs[83] concludes that a number of assessment tools are appropriate for use with cognitively impaired older adults, but makes no reference to how reliable they are. However, she does suggest that the assessor should take time to decide which tool is the most appropriate to use for an individual patient. However, one could surmise that if this is done, then a tool or scale will be selected on the basis of whether it supports the nurse's observations, rather than the patient's actual experience of pain, as the nurse may select a tool to justify a subjective bias.

It is clear that there will be difficulties in finding a reliable instrument for the assessment of pain in the older adult who cannot communicate effectively. Simons and Malabar[81] have discounted several tools because they fail to differentiate between expressions of discomfort (e.g. reactions to environmental stimuli such as excessive environmental noise) and pain. Instruments used for assessing pain in children were discounted because although demented adults may exhibit some of the same behavioural traits as children, these instruments had not been tested for their reliability in adults. Simons and Malabar[81] also cite difficulties in differentiating between pain and the manifestations of depression. If this presents problems with assessing pain, it may also mean that depression will remain unrecognised.

A reliable assessment may not always be possible due to variations in a patient's condition over a specified period of time, and nurses and other healthcare workers may not always recognise and respond to changes in the patient's condition.[55] Huffman and Kunik[87] reiterate the importance of further research into the assessment of pain in cognitively impaired older adults. There are disparities in the treatment of pain in a group for whom the incidence of pain is thought to be high. A lack of investigation and thus understanding of the cognitive experience of pain in this group further complicate the issue of assessment.[87]

Informal caregivers: the reliability of their information

As the number of beds available in residential care homes continues to fall,[88] there will be an increasing reliance on the care provided by family and other informal carers of older adults. Although the patient should always be regarded as the primary source of information, it may not always be possible for them to provide this, and nurses may find information provided by informal caregivers useful. However, they should be aware both that this information might be unreliable, and that by seeking it they may be compromising the patient's right to privacy (*see* Chapter 7). Discrepancies in information provided by patients and their informal caregivers may be either intentional or unintentional. For example, Trapp-Moen *et al.*[89] suggest that 'erroneous descriptions of an individual's abilities [by a relative] may occur because of ignorance, or fear of a nursing home placement' (p. 406).

Research by Feinberg and Whitlatch[66] found some discrepancy between the informal caregiver's and care receiver's responses to questions about the patient's demographic details, preferences and choices. Although this might be due to the care receivers providing an incorrect response as a result of their cognitive impairment, it could equally well be due to the informal caregiver's lack of knowledge about the care receiver. This has important implications for nurses who may rely on information provided by informal caregivers when assessing cognitively impaired patients. One of the questions that provoked incongruent responses asked informal caregivers how many children the care receiver had. It is certainly not beyond the realms of possibility that the patient may have children of whom their other children or spouse are unaware. Remember that even as recently as the 1980s there was some social stigma attached to raising a child outside wedlock. During the war, many men went away for months or years, or never returned home. If children were conceived during these absences, it is possible that their mothers would surrender them for adoption rather than have to make some very difficult explanations and meet with the disapproval of their community. In such cases their siblings would have been unaware of their existence.

Returning to the study, interestingly the criteria for sample selection stated that the caregiver should be a spouse or adult child of the care receiver, but the researchers did not appear to consider the possibility that some members of this group, of which more than 50% were over 65 years of age, might be suffering from some degree of cognitive impairment themselves (*see* p. 84). The researchers also gave no indication of how the accuracy of the responses to the baseline questions was verified. Did they simply accept the response of the caregivers as being the truth? For this reason, nurses should also exercise caution when there is a discrepancy between the information provided by the patient and their family or friends.

Research also indicates some lack of agreement between the evaluation by informal caregivers and by the patient (both demented and non-demented) of the patient's ability to perform the activities of daily living.[90] It could be argued that if the patient is capable of providing an evaluation of their own ability to perform activities, then there should be no reason to consult informal caregivers for this information, and certainly not without the patient's consent (*see* Chapter 7).

Although Nolan *et al.*[91] advocate that informal carers should be considered as co-workers who are valued and involved in the care process, the nurse should also exercise caution when considering the information provided by these informal caregivers. As already mentioned, many informal carers of older adults are themselves elderly.[92] It may be that the assumption of a caring role has evolved from a long, loving and caring relationship with the patient, and the caregiver is well intentioned and a source of invaluable information. However, some relatives may reluctantly take on the care of someone with whom they have had an unhappy relationship.[92]

Whatever the basis of the carer role, tensions may exist between informal carers and healthcare professionals. The informal carer may feel that nurses expect too much of them, and that they are being unfairly burdened, or conversely they may consider interventions by nurses to be unwelcome and an invasion of privacy.[92] There is also a possibility that informal caregivers may collaborate with those they are caring for – for example, in denial of a loved one's increasing dependence.[93,94] (Recall the example of Fred and Vera Atkins on p. 77.[93,94]) Collusion may be intentional or unintentional, for reasons already outlined. Eventually the informal carer may find that they are no longer able to cope. Their response to this situation may be overt or covert requests for help, or a sense of guilt may drive them to struggle on alone.

The interaction between nurse and patient

The demeanour and conduct of the patient may influence the nurse's perception and therefore their assessment of that patient (*see* Chapter 5). They may be quiet and uncomplaining or loud and demanding, and a nurse may misinterpret what is an actual need as laziness or unco-operativeness. However, regardless of its basis, a need is a need. An individual will experience satisfaction when their needs are fulfilled, but tensions will arise if they are not.[95] These tensions may manifest themselves in many ways – for example, as aggression or social withdrawal.

Perceptions of what is deviant or difficult behaviour are usually subjective and may depend on the individuals involved (both staff and patient) and the context of the behaviour (*see* Chapter 5). Stockwell,[96] in her writings on *The Unpopular Patient*, postulates that individuals operating as a group are bound by implicit and explicit rules governing behaviour. If a member of the group does not abide by these rules, then other group members will consider them 'deviant' and they will become unpopular. Such contentious activities may include making what are considered to be excessive demands on the nurses' time, aggressive or confrontational behaviour, not doing enough to help oneself, and having what is deemed to be a self-inflicted illness or injury. The nurse may lose their ability to view the patient and their needs objectively, and future interactions with the patient may therefore be prejudiced.

When nurses are busy or emotionally stressed, they may lack the patience necessary to cope with a patient's demands,[97] and this cycle of events may also work in the other direction. Nurses themselves may become unpopular with patients, and if they are perceived to be unsympathetic or uncaring this will influence how the patient responds to them. Indeed, a study by Patterson[98] examined a sample of 12 nursing home patients' perceptions of supportive and non-supportive behaviour in nurses. The findings indicate that patients rate nurses who display negative attitudes towards them, or who fail to demonstrate respect or concern, as non-supportive.

Hornby[99] explains that patients very quickly recognise 'good nurses' – those who respond to them as valued individuals and respect their needs. Watson's *Philosophy and Science of Caring*[100] acknowledges the satisfaction experienced by both nurse and patient when a trusting interpersonal relationship is established. This is a humanistic approach to nursing, and it supports Peplau's assertion that humans strive for a sense of security and satisfaction, and that behaviour is driven by this desire.[95] Burnard argues that nurses care for others because they must.[101] Those who are driven to care recognise their own humanity and the humanity of others, and thus the need to care for others as we would expect to be cared for ourselves. However, in order to respect an individual's humanity there is first a need for acceptance of both positive and negative feelings within the relationship. If this acceptance is not reached, then a mutually satisfying relationship will not be achieved, and the patient will not receive unconditional regard.

Olsen[102] suggests that the essence of a patient's humanity, and therefore personhood, is the creation of meaning for their individual world. Although all individuals have such creation of meaning in common, it is likely that the content will be different. Olsen asserts that the basis of a nurse's empathy for their patients will be the recognition that patients may choose to live their life in their own different ways, and take risks and adopt behaviours of which the nurse may not approve. The nurse will acknowledge the fact that this represents an individual patient's personhood and their right to choice.

Olsen[102] also explores the concept of empathetic maturity and proposes that the greater the empathetic maturity, the higher that person's level of moral reasoning (*see* Chapter 7). This will enable a greater consideration of others as people, and attribution of greater value to the concept of personhood. Those with a less developed empathetic maturity are likely to be influenced by factors such as the degree to which they perceive the patient to be responsible for their own condition, and the extent to which they approve of their lifestyle. This will affect the way in which the nurse relates to the patient. But how does this relate to assessment? A nurse who is unable to recognise and therefore value the personhood of a patient with severe cognitive impairment is unlikely to make an accurate holistic assessment of their status. Such cognitive impairment may restrict an individual's ability to make and communicate choices, to comprehend fully their situation and to store and retrieve information.[103] The empathy of nurses, and evaluation of what is significant and important in the patient's life, are necessary if the patient's personhood is to be recognised and acknowledged in the assessment of needs and provision of care.

Research by Haggstrom and Norberg[104] investigated factors identified as being integral to the provision of 'good' care for people with dementia. Although there are limitations associated with the method of sample selection, the findings are interesting. They indicate that the characteristics of 'good' care include having a positive regard for the patient's history and encompassing this in nursing care, making a consistent effort to facilitate two-way communication, and being aware of changes in the patient's state and responding to them with understanding. Such attributes may be especially important when considering the difficulties encountered when caring for individuals with dementia,[105] who may exhibit behaviour that does not conform to social norms, and who may have high levels of dependency and problems with communication. A study by Beck[106] investigated nursing students' experiences of caring for older adults with cognitive impairment. The findings indeed suggest that students consider empathy to be instrumental in coping with the psychological and physical demands of caring for people with dementia, but that this empathy only develops as they get to know the patient.

Another study explored the effects on the status of dementia sufferers in a nursing home of shifting from a task-centred approach to care to a more client-centred approach. The findings indicate that adopting a more client-centred approach may result in residents being less verbally aggressive and staff reporting lower stress levels. Although the findings cannot be generalised, one could infer that the two outcomes are related, and that as staff become less preoccupied with completing tasks and more responsive to their patients, they develop a greater understanding of their patients' needs.[107]

It is clear that in order for a nurse to provide effective care for an individual with dementia, they will need to have a good understanding of both the patient's current status and their history. The nurse will need to establish what is important to the patient and what makes them the person that they are. Such recognition of patients as individuals has been shown to benefit them in a study by Bourgeouis et al.[108] Davies et al.,[23] in their review of the literature concerning the relationship between communication, the promotion of autonomy and independence, suggest that the quality of communication between the nurse and their patient will influence the quality of care delivered. The nurse needs to understand what makes the patient happy and what causes them distress. For example, aggressive behaviours are often exhibited when a patient with dementia is hurried,[94] but nurses may attribute this to other causes, and may fail to acknowledge their own contribution to this behaviour. Furthermore, the distress of patients with dementia may manifest itself in many different ways.[94] Unfortunately, the findings of Davies et al.[23] suggest that an understanding of patient reactions might be difficult to achieve. This is because they found that the majority of interactions between nurses and their older patients are short, directed by the nurse and usually connected with task completion rather than with nurse motivation to develop a greater understanding of the patient. There is indeed a danger that accommodation of physical needs will become the focus for care.[109]

It is clear that those caring for older adults should be able to demonstrate a positive attitude to both the patients and their care,[110] and an understanding of their specific problems and needs, if a valid and reliable assessment is to be made. Unfortunately, this is often not the case, with old age popularly being conceptualised as a stage of decline and decay that is merely a preparation for death.[111] Nurses may lack the patience, time and motivation to understand their patients and the way they behave.

In summary

This review of the literature explores the many and complex ways in which the nurse, the patient and other healthcare professionals interact during the assessment and care process. Most significantly it highlights the many ways in which the efficacy of the assessment process may be compromised. The need for the nurse who is making the assessment to be committed to facilitating the patient's contribution to this process is highlighted.

If the nurse is unaware of the needs of the patient, is insensitive to the special requirements that older people may have, or is generally unsympathetic, then an effective assessment may not be effected. If the individual who is being assessed is unwilling or unable to contribute to the process, the information that is made available to the nurse will be compromised, and the nurse will be dependent upon information from other healthcare workers and the patient's informal carers. The various ways in which this information might be flawed have been demonstrated.

Key points

- Decisions and judgements are based on information from a variety of sources.
- Nurses often rely on information obtained from themselves and other people, rather than from other sources, such as research or audits.
- Any inaccuracies in this information will impair the quality of the assessment. There are a number of different ways in which the quality of an assessment may be compromised.
  - Nurses may lack the skills, knowledge and/or experience necessary to recognise and acknowledge relevant changes in a patient's condition.
  - Despite a clear need to involve patients in the assessment process, patients may find it difficult to communicate their needs because of cognitive impairment or because they are experiencing difficulties with communication.
  - Nurses may find it difficult to involve patients with communication difficulties or cognitive impairment in the assessment process, and some patients may be inappropriately excluded from the process.
  - Nurses may find it difficult to remember that their very frail and dependent patients were once independent beings, and that the person they once were still exists and should be acknowledged.
  - Patients may be unused to participating in decisions relating to their healthcare, and find it difficult to do this.
  - Patients may be reluctant to discuss their needs because of embarrassment.
  - Patients may be reluctant to discuss their needs because they fear dependency, and are afraid of being admitted to a nursing home or hospital.
  - Nurses may not give their patients the time, support and privacy necessary to encourage their participation in the assessment process.
  - Informal caregivers may be an unreliable source of information.

References

1   Carnwell R (2000) Essential differences between research and evidence-based practice. *Nurse Res.* **8:** 55–68.

2   Thompson C (2002) The value of research in clinical decision making. *Nurs Times.* **98:** 30–4.

3   Estabrooks CA *et al.* (2003) Individual determinants of research utilisation: a systematic review. *J Adv Nurs.* **43**: 506–20.
4   Fulbrook P (2003) Developing best practice in critical care nursing: knowledge, evidence and practice. *Nurs Crit Care.* **8**: 96–102.
5   Jolley S (2002) Raising research awareness: a strategy for nurses. *Nurs Standard.* **16**: 33–9.
6   Halstead T (2002) Using research to improve a ward-based learning environment. *Nurs Times.* **98**: 36.
7   Breen A (2002) How research helps nurses learn from patients with dementia. *Nurs Times.* **98**: 33.
8   Freeman J (2002) Dealing with drugs in acute psychiatry: knowing the score. *Ment Health Pract.* **5**: 18–22.
9   Lefler L (2002) Evidence-based practice. The advanced nurse's role regarding women's delay in seeking treatment with myocardial infarction. *J Am Acad Nurse Pract.* **14**: 449–56.
10 Australian National Institute of Clinical Studies (ANICS) (2003) *Information Finding and Assessment Methods that Different Groups of Clinicians Find Most Useful.* Prepared by the Centre for Clinical Effectiveness, ANICS, Melbourne.
11 Thompson C *et al.* (2001) The accessibility of research-based knowledge for nurses in United Kingdom acute care settings. *J Adv Nurs.* **36**: 11–22.
12 McWilliam S (2003) The research practice gap in radiotherapy. *Synergy.* **July:** 7–10.
13 Corlett J *et al.* (2003) Factors influencing theoretical knowledge and practical skill acquisition in student nurses: an empirical experiment. *Nurse Educ Today.* **23**: 183–90.
14 Landers M (2001) The theory/practice gap in nursing: the view of the students. *All Ireland J Nurs Midwifery.* **1**: 142–7.
15 Kerrison S, Clarke A and Doehr S (1999) People and paper: information for evidence-based practice and the differing needs of doctors and nurses. *J Interprof Care.* **13**: 289–99.
16 Colley S (2003) Nursing theory: its importance to practice. *Nurs Standard.* **17**: 33–7.
17 Giuliano KK (2003) Expanding the use of empiricism in nursing: can we bridge the gap between knowledge and clinical practice? *Nurs Philosophy.* **4**: 44–52.
18 Seymour B, Kinn S and Sutherland N (2003) Valuing both critical and creative thinking in clinical practice: narrowing the research–practice gap? *J Adv Nurs.* **42**: 288–96.
19 McCleary L and Brown GT (2003) Barriers to paediatric nurses' research utilisation. *J Adv Nurs.* **42**: 364–72.
20 Taylor H (2003a) It's not what you do – it's the way that you do it. *Nursing Older People.* **14**: 32.
21 Holden U (ed.) (1988) *Neuropsychology and Ageing: definitions, explanations and practical approaches.* Croom Helm, London.
22 Blakemore K and Drake RF (1996) *Understanding Equal Opportunities Policies.* Prentice Hall, Hemel Hempstead.
23 Davies S, Laker S and Ellis L (1997) Promoting autonomy and independence for older people within nursing practice: a literature review. *J Adv Nurs.* **26**: 408–17.
24 Baltes MM (1996) *The Many Faces of Dependency in Old Age.* Cambridge University Press, Cambridge.
25 Heath H (2000) Assessing older people. *Elderly Care.* **11**: 27–8.
26 Cioffi J (1998) Decision making by emergency nurses in triage assessments. *Accid Emerg Nurs.* **6**: 184–91.
27 Tanner CA *et al.* (1987) Diagnostic reasoning strategies of nurses and nursing students. *Nurs Res.* **36**: 358–63.
28 Corcoran S (1986) Task complexity and nursing expertise as factors in decision making. *Nurs Res.* **35**: 107–12.

29 Prescott PA, Soeken KL and Ryan JW (1989) Measuring patient intensity: a reliability study. *Eval Health Prof.* **12:** 255–69.

30 Aggleton P and Chalmers H (2000) *Nursing Models and Nursing Practice* (2e). Macmillan, Basingstoke.

31 Department of Health (2001) *National Service Framework for Older People.* Department of Health, London.

32 Rodwell CM (1996) An analysis of the concept of empowerment. *J Adv Nurs.* **23:** 305–13.

33 Department of Health (1995) *The Community Care Act.* HMSO, London.

34 Caldock K (1993) A preliminary study of changes in assessment: examining the relationship between recent policy and practitioners' knowledge, opinions and practice. *Health Soc Care.* **1:** 139–46.

35 Department of Health (1989) *Caring for People: community care in the next decade and beyond.* HMSO, London.

36 Backett K and Davison C (1992) Rational or reasonable? Perceptions of health at different stages of life. *Health Educ J.* **51:** 55–9.

37 Sherbourne CD *et al.* (1999) Relationship between age and patients' current health state preferences. *Gerontologist.* **39:** 271–8.

38 Lawton MP *et al.* (1999) Health, valuation of life, and the wish to live. *Gerontologist.* **39:** 406–16.

39 Stuart-Hamilton I (2000) *The Psychology of Ageing: an introduction* (3e). Jessica Kingsley Publishers, London.

40 Scrutton S (1990) Ageism: the foundation of age discrimination. In: E McEwen (ed.) *Age: the unrecognised discrimination.* Age Concern, London.

41 Baker DI *et al.* (2001) The design and implementation of a restorative care model for home care. *Gerontologist.* **41:** 257–63.

42 Webster C (1991) The elderly and the early National Health Service. In: M Pelling and RM Smith (eds) *Life, Death and the Elderly: historical perspectives.* Routledge, London.

43 Simmons SF and Schnelle JF (1999) Strategies to measure nursing home residents' satisfaction and preferences related to incontinence and mobility care: implications for evaluating intervention effects. *Gerontologist.* **39:** 345–55.

44 Carpenter BD *et al.* (2000) The psychosocial preferences of older adults: a pilot examination of content and structure. *Gerontologist.* **40:** 335–48.

45 Bowers BJ, Fibich B and Jacobson N (2001) Care-as-service, care-as-relating, care-as-comfort: understanding nursing home residents' definitions of quality. *Gerontologist.* **41:** 539–45.

46 Hansen T *et al.* (2002) Discrepancies between patients and professionals in the assessment of patient needs: a quantitative study of Norwegian mental health care. *J Adv Nurs.* **39:** 554–62.

47 Hudson KA and Sexton DL (1996) Perceptions about nursing care: comparing elders' and nurses' priorities. *J Gerontol Nurs.* **22** (12): 41–6.

48 Pearson A *et al.* (1993) Quality of care in nursing homes: from the resident's perspective. *J Adv Nurs.* **18:** 20–4.

49 *The Observer* (2002) 50 years of 'opening-up': 1952-2002.. 27 October. www.observer.guardian.co.uk/sex/story/0.12550.818309.00.html (last accessed 19 May 2005)

50 Buffam H *et al.* (1928) *Virtue's Household Physician: a twentieth-century Medica.* Virtue and Company Ltd, London.

51 Chur-Hansen A (2002) Preference for female and male nurses: the role of age, gender and previous experience. *J Adv Nurs.* **37:** 192–8.

52 Bowling A (1995) *Measuring Disease.* Open University Press, Buckingham.

53 Chiriboga DA, McHugh D and Sweeney MA (2004) The Mini-Mental Exam (Mini-ME): an unobtrusive and brief test for cognitive problems? *Clin Gerontologist.* **27:** 3–13.

54 Bowling A (1997) *Research Methods in Health: investigating health and health services.* Open University Press, Buckingham.

55 Hawes C *et al.* (1995) Reliability estimates for the minimum data set for nursing home resident assessment and care screening (MDS). *Gerontologist.* **35:** 172–8.

56 Hybels CF, Blazer DG and Pieper CF (2001) Toward a threshold for subthreshold depression: an analysis of correlates of depression by severity of symptoms using data from an elderly community sample. *Gerontologist.* **41:** 357–65.

57 Loeher KE *et al.* (2004) Nursing home transition and depressive symptoms in older medical rehabilitation patients. *Clin Gerontologist.* **27:** 59–70.

58 Bischkopf J, Busse A and Angermeyer MC (2002) Mild cognitive impairment – a review of prevalence, incidence and outcome according to current approaches. *Acta Psychiatr Scand.* **106:** 403–14.

59 Tait C and Fuller E (2002) *Health Survey for England 2000: psychosocial well-being among older people.* The Stationery Office, London.

60 Hanninen T *et al.* (2002) Prevalence of mild cognitive impairment: a population-based study in elderly subjects. *Acta Neurol Scand.* **106:** 148–54.

61 Evans O *et al.* (2003) *The Mental Health of Older People.* The Stationery Office, London.

62 Magaziner J *et al.* (2000) The prevalence of dementia in a state-wide sample of new nursing home admissions aged 65 and older: diagnosis by expert panel. *Gerontologist.* **40:** 663–72.

63 Keady J and Bender MP (1998) Changing faces: the purpose and practice of assessing older adults with cognitive impairment. *Health Care Later Life.* **3:** 129–44.

64 Storey JE *et al.* (2004) The Rowlands Universal Dementia Assessment Scale (RUDAS): a multicultural cognitive assessment scale. *Int Psychogeriatrics.* **16:** 13–31.

65 Sansone P *et al.* (1998) Determining the capacity of demented nursing home residents to name a health care proxy. *Clin Gerontologist.* **19:** 35–50.

66 Feinberg LF and Whitlatch CJ (2001) Are persons with cognitive impairment able to state consistent choices? *Gerontologist.* **41:** 374–82.

67 Moye J *et al.* (2004) Capacity to consent to treatment: empirical comparison of three instruments in older adults with and without dementia. *Gerontologist.* **44:** 166–75.

68 Simmons SF and Schnelle JF (2001) The identification of residents capable of accurately describing daily care: implications for evaluating nursing home care quality. *Gerontologist.* **41:** 605–11.

69 Pearson A *et al.* (1993) Quality of care in nursing homes: from the resident's perspective. *J Adv Nurs.* **18:** 20–4.

70 Wahl H-W, Oswald F and Zimprich D (1999) Everyday competence in visually impaired older adults: a case for person–environment perspectives. *Gerontologist.* **39:** 140–9.

71 Strawbridge WJ *et al.* (2000) Negative consequences of hearing impairment in old age: a longitudinal analysis. *Gerontologist.* **40:** 320–6.

72 Brennan M and Cardinali G (2000) The use of pre-existing and novel coping strategies in adapting to age-related vision loss. *Gerontologist.* **40:** 327–34.

73 Hemsley B *et al.* (2001) Nursing the patient with severe communication impairment. *J Adv Nurs.* **35:** 827–35.

74 Hines J (1997) Making the right noises: caring for hearing-impaired patients. *Nurs Times.* **93:** 31–3.

75 Horn S and Munafo M (1997) *Pain: theory, research and intervention.* Open University Press, Buckingham.

76 Melzack R and Wall P (1996) *The Challenge of Pain.* Penguin, New York.

77 Helman CG (1994) *Culture, Health and Illness* (3e). Butterworth-Heinemann, Oxford.

78 Gehring M and Watson R (1999) Chronic pain in the elderly. *Elderly Care.* **11:** 16–20.

79 Hayes R (1995) Pain assessment in the elderly. *Br J Nurs.* **4** (20): 1199–204.

80 Ferrell BA, Ferrell BR and Osterweil D (1990) Pain in the nursing home. *J Am Geriatr Soc.* **38:** 409–14.

81 Simons W and Malabar R (1995) Assessing pain in elderly patients who cannot respond verbally. *J Adv Nurs.* **22:** 663–9.

82 Camp DL (1987) Comparison of medical, surgical and oncology patients' descriptions of pain and nurses' documentation of pain assessments. *J Adv Nurs.* **12:** 593–8.

83 Briggs E (2001) Principles of pain assessment in older people. Part 2. *Nursing Older People.* **13:** 27–8.

84 Zwakhalen SMG *et al.* (2004) Pain assessment in intellectually disabled people: non-verbal indicators. *J Adv Nurs.* **45:** 236–45.

85 Fries BE *et al.* (2001) Pain in US nursing homes: validating a pain scale for the minimum data set. *Gerontologist.* **41:** 173–9.

86 Wynne CF, Ling SM and Remsburg R (2000) Comparison of pain assessment instruments in cognitively intact and cognitively impaired nursing home residents. *Geriatr Nurs.* **21:** 20–3.

87 Huffman JC and Kunik ME (2000) Assessment and understanding of pain in patients with dementia. *Gerontologist.* **40:** 574–81.

88 National Statistics (2004) *Places Available in Residential Care Homes: by type of care home, at 31 March 2001. Regional Trends 37;* www.statistics.gov.uk/StatBase/Expodata/spreadsheets/D5947.xls

89 Trap-Moen B *et al.* (2001) In-home assessment of dementia by nurses: experience using the CERAD evaluations. *Gerontologist.* **41:** 406–9.

90 Ostbye T *et al.* (1997) Reported activities of daily living: agreement between elderly subjects with and without dementia and their caregivers. *Age Ageing.* **26:** 99–106.

91 Nolan M and Caldock K (1996) Assessment: identifying the barriers to good practice. *Health Soc Care Commun.* **4:** 77–85.

92 National Statistics (2001) *The Offical Yearbook of Great Britain and Northern Ireland.* The Stationery Office, London.

93 Fish S (1997) *Alzheimer's* (4e). Lion Publishing, Oxford.

94 Murphy E (1986) *Dementia and Mental Illness in the Old.* Papermac, London.

95 Peplau H (1988) *Interpersonal Relations in Nursing.* Macmillan, London.

96 Stockwell F (1972) *The Unpopular Patient.* Royal College of Nursing, London.

97 Bond M (1986) *Stress and Self-Awareness: a guide for nurses.* Heinemann Nursing, Oxford.

98 Patterson BJ (1995) The process of social support: adjusting to life in a nursing home. *J Adv Nurs.* **21:** 682–9.

99 Hornby M (2002) Total courage. *Nurs Times.* **98:** 24–5.

100 Watson J (1989) Philosophy and science of caring. In: A Marriner-Tomey (ed.) *Nursing Theorists and Their Work.* CV Mosby Company, St Louis, MO.

101 Burnard P (1997) Why care? Ethical and spiritual issues in caring nursing. In: G Brykczynska (ed.) *Caring: the compassion and wisdom of nursing.* Edward Arnold, London.

102 Olsen DP (1997) Development of an instrument to measure the cognitive structure used to understand personhood in patients. *Nurs Res.* **46:** 78–84.

103 Powers BA (2001) Ethnographic analysis of everyday ethics in the care of nursing home residents with dementia: taxonomy. *Nurs Res.* **50:** 332–9.

104 Haggstrom T and Norberg A (1996) Maternal thinking in dementia care. *J Adv Nurs.* **24:** 431–8.

105 Ballard C *et al.* (2001) Quality of care in private sector and NHS facilities for people with dementia: cross-sectional survey. *BMJ.* **323:** 426–7.

106 Beck CT (1996) Nursing students' experiences caring for cognitively impaired older people. *J Adv Nurs.* **23:** 992–8.

107 Matthews EA, Farrell GA and Blackmore AM (1996) Effects of an environmental

manipulation emphasising client-centred care on agitation and sleep in dementia sufferers in a nursing home. *J Adv Nurs*. **24:** 439–47.

108 Bourgeois MS *et al.* (2004) Communication skills training for nursing aides of residents with dementia: the impact of measuring performance. *Clin Gerontologist*. **27:** 119–38.

109 Jenkins D and Price B (1996) Dementia and personhood: a focus for care? *J Adv Nurs*. **24:** 84–90.

110 United Kingdom Central Council (UKCC) (1997) *The Nursing and Health Visiting Contribution to the Continuing Care of Older People*. UKCC, London.

111 Elliott G (2000) *'Teach Granny too.' Images of ageing: towards a contemporary theory of lifespan development*. Paper presented at the British Educational Research Association Conference, University of Cardiff, 7–10 September.

Chapter 7

Ethical, professional and legal requirements to involve older adults in decisions about their care

Introduction

Chapter 4 considered how decisions are made as part of the assessment process. Information-processing theory, intuition and the cognitive continuum theory were examined, and it has been established that regardless of the decision-making model adopted, nurses will already have obtained or will need to acquire information from somewhere if they are going to be able to make an informed decision about their patient.

Patient autonomy and freedom to choose

In an ideal world, the patient him- or herself would be directly involved in the decision-making process. Decisions relating to patients involve the patient, and should in most cases be informed by the patient and their preferences. However, there may be circumstances where it is not possible for the patient to be actively involved in decision making. In situations such as these, nurses will need to obtain information from other sources. However, there may be circumstances where the patient is excluded from the assessment process inappropriately (*see* Chapter 6), usually because the nurse regards them as incapable of participating or providing valid information. Yet there is strong evidence that even individuals with cognitive impairments can and should be involved in decisions relating to their care and treatment (*see* Chapters 6 and 7), and it is important that nurses are aware of this if they are to provide truly patient-centred care.

Regardless of the patient's cognitive state or the way in which they behave, nurses should remember to have respect for the patient as a person, and endeavour to understand what is important to them. Nurses have responsibilities to patients at both a professional and a human level. Nursing is a humane profession that requires the recognition of a patient's humanity, regardless of their behaviour or appearance, and their need to be treated as we would hope to be treated ourselves,[1] with dignity.[2]

But why is all of this so important? It has been acknowledged that maintaining patient dignity is an essential feature of nursing care, and research conducted by Walsh and Kowanko[3] found that although patient and nurse perceptions of dignity varied slightly, characteristics common to both groups were respect, privacy and control. It is difficult to feel dignified if our wishes are ignored, and our right to live our life in the manner of our choice is not acknowledged.

You walk on to the ward, hesitant and afraid. Your husband grips your elbow reassuringly, and you smile at him in gratitude. A group of nurses, clearly very busy, are huddled by the nurses' station. You stand next to them for a few moments, but no one seems to notice that you are there. Suddenly one of them looks up, and asks no one in particular – 'Ethel Jones?' You nod – words of agreement don't seem to want to come out. You realise that the nurse is looking at your husband. 'Mrs Jones?', she asks him again. He tells her that yes, this is Mrs Jones. She gestures for you to follow, and is already halfway down the ward before she realises that you do not move quite as quickly as she does. When you eventually reach her, she gestures to a chair, looks at your husband again and tells him that he should get you settled and unpack your belongings. She makes to leave the bedside, but thinks again, and looks down at the bundle of notes she is holding. 'Your wife, Mr Jones, it says here that she has Alzheimer's', she says without looking up. 'Will you be staying with her for a bit, you know, help us fill in some of the paperwork?' Without giving your husband a chance to say a word, never mind you, she dashes off. She has not yet made eye contact with you.

How do you imagine that you would feel in these circumstances? Angry, humiliated and afraid? There has been no acknowledgement of you as a person, just as a patient on a list, with just one word predetermining how that nurse would behave towards you.

'Empowerment' is a term frequently used in both nursing theory and practice,[4] and although there is some variation in its definition, it generally refers to the process of facilitating a client's autonomy.[5] Patients may be 'encouraged to take responsibility for their own health and decisions concerning their life'[6] (p. 75) if nurses work to promote their self-esteem and sense of value. However, this will only be possible if the nurse is first able to accept that the patient's decisions may have a negative effect on their health.[6] Chapter 6 considered the possibility that the patient and the nurse or other healthcare professional may have different expectations of healthcare. If they have grown up in the UK, older people may not expect to be involved in decisions relating to their healthcare for two main reasons. First, they have experienced a healthcare system in which there was very little patient participation in choosing between limited healthcare options (*see* Chapter 6). Second, in the past there has been a paternalistic approach to healthcare where it has been accepted that the expert knowledge and experience of practitioners best equips them to make decisions and choices on the patient's behalf.[7]

Paternalism may be 'strong' in circumstances where the practitioner makes a choice about treatment without even consulting the patient, or it may be more subtle if the patient is presented with a choice, but given biased or limited information which would prompt selection of the option favoured by the practitioner.[7] It may be difficult for patients to participate in healthcare decisions if they have not previously been encouraged to do so. It is therefore possible that these people will still expect doctors and nurses to make decisions on their behalf, in accordance with the paternalistic approach to care that historically was the accepted practice.

Ageism

The concept of ageism has been explored in Chapter 5. Treating someone differently on the basis of their age alone would constitute an ageist act. Nurses must be careful that neither a patient's age nor the manifestations of the ageing process detract from the patient's right to be treated as an autonomous being. The government has declared its lack of tolerance of ageism, and its respect for the differing needs and requirements of different groups in society:[8]

> The NHS of the twenty-first century must be responsive to the needs of different groups and individuals within society and challenge discrimination on the grounds of age, gender, ethnicity, religion, disability and sexuality. The NHS will treat patients as individuals, with respect for their dignity.   (p. 4)

Although there is no specific legislation protecting against ageism,[9] an individual nurse's behaviour will usually be determined by their morals and ethics and by the law, and their professional behaviour will be dictated by codes of professional conduct and by personal and societal expectations of the nurse's role (*see* Chapter 3). These are encompassed by the laws and ethical codes which dictate standards of professional conduct. There is a strong ethical, professional and legal impetus for the nurse to make every effort to involve their older patients in assessment and decision making.

Perceptions and expectations of the nurse role were examined in Chapter 3. It is now necessary to consider ethical, professional and legal obligations in more depth. Although these three areas are considered as separate entities here, in practice, ethics and the law are often inextricably interlinked and entwined within the *Code of Professional Conduct*.[10,11]

Ethical requirements

Ethics are often referred to in relation to nurses' practice, and have been described as fundamental to the practice of nursing.[12] But what are ethics? Burkhardt and Nathaniel[13] describe ethics as 'a formal process for making logical and consistent decisions based upon moral beliefs' (p. 420), with 'morals' constituting the general description of 'the standards of behaviour actually held or followed by individuals and particular groups of people'[14] (p. 16). The terms 'ethics' and 'morals' are often used interchangeably, and tend to refer to a philosophical framework that guides individuals and groups in their pursuit of 'doing the right thing'.

References to ethics may relate to what ought to be 'inquiry that attempts to answer the question "Which general norms for the guidance and evaluation of conduct are worthy of moral acceptance?"(normative) or how things actually are (descriptive)'[15] (p. 4). The *Code of Professional Conduct*[11] outlines the normative code of ethics for nurses. A number of ethical theories provide a framework that may assist in the evaluation of actions and judgements.[15] Those considered most influential in moral reasoning might be broadly grouped into two categories, namely consequentialism and deontology.[14]

Consequentialist theory

This is concerned with the consequences of an action or series of actions, rather than with the act itself. The first requirement is to determine what would be the 'best outcome'. The 'best act' would therefore be the one that would be necessary to achieve that outcome. *Utilitarianism* is a consequentialist theory 'concerned with acts which enable the greatest good for the greatest number of people'[12] (p. 4). An example of a utilitarian perspective would be the allocation of healthcare resources. A utilitarian would consider it ethically wrong to invest in highly expensive surgery to benefit one patient, at the expense of treatment that would make a difference to the lives of hundreds of others.

Non-consequentialist theory

The predominant non-consequentialist theory is *deontology*, which considers that the act is more important than the outcome. Doing the 'right thing' matters, and the consequences of that action have no ethical relevance – the good is in the fulfilment of the duty.[12] In the example given in the previous section, the 'right act' would be to treat the patient, regardless of the financial cost. If the treatment is available, and it will help to ease the patient's suffering, then it should be given. The actual or potential outcomes (i.e. potentially depriving perhaps hundreds of other patients of healthcare resources) are seen as irrelevant. Immanuel Kant (1724–1804), a Prussian philosopher, is perhaps the best-known deontologist.[13–17] He advocated his belief in living according to moral rules that were termed the *Categorical Imperative*: 'Act only according to that maxim by which you can at the same time will that it should become a universal law'.

For example, if one decides that it is wrong to lie, then it is always wrong to lie.[16] The emphasis of deontology is on the equality and autonomy of individuals. Kant's practical imperative states: 'Act so that you treat humanity, whether in your own person or that of another, always as an end and never as a means only'[13] (p. 32).

This means that individuals should work in partnership with others in order to fulfil duties to them.[13] There is a recognition that it is morally wrong to strive for a particular outcome at the expense of the individuals involved.[12]

Criticisms of ethical theories

Although these are only very brief overviews of ethical theory, they do give some insight into different ways of viewing 'doing the right thing'. However, it can also be seen that ethical theories are abstract concepts, which may present problems if directly applied to practice. Examples in relation to consequentialism, utilitarianism and deontology are listed below.

Consequentialism

- Who decides what is a 'good' outcome?[7]

Utilitarianism

A number of points have been raised in relation to utilitarian theory.[16]

- The nurse's main responsibility is to provide individualised care, and the patient has the right to choose their own options. Utilitarianism would deny this right.
- If the theory directs attention to the consequences of the nurse's action, are the patient's thoughts, feelings and perspectives being taken into account?
- If the nurse's main responsibility is to provide individualised care, then surely the patient has the right to determine their own outcomes? Utilitarian theory would deny this right.
- Is the person who is deciding what is 'good' the one with the most power?[17]
- The greatest good for the majority may not be the greatest good for the individual.

Deontology

- It is difficult to see how it is feasible for nurses to act without thinking of the consequences of their actions.
- The purpose of the moral rule is only the rule itself.[16]
- It is the quality of a nurse's decisions that are important, and not the effect that they may have on the patient. There is a disregard of patient uniqueness and autonomy.[16]
- There is no differentiation between harm and benefit.[16]
- If nurses are to live and act by moral rules, then it is difficult to see how they could support the freedom and autonomy of a patient who wishes to live by what the nurse may consider to be immoral standards. If the nurse was to support these actions, they would be neglecting their actions.[16]
- The rules are inflexible, but each patients is different, and a rule that may be applicable to one may not be applicable to all.[15]

Ethical principles

It is clear that although the ethical theories may provide a useful contribution to moral reasoning, they may be too abstract to apply rigidly to the diverse situations that are encountered daily by nurses. However, a number of general principles have been derived from these ethical theories, and these may be of more use and applicability in relation to the justification of a nurse's actions and behaviours.[14] Singleton and McLaren[7] have outlined four philosophical principles which may be used when considering ethical issues:

- the principle of autonomy – the individual has a right to be self-governing
- the principle of beneficence – the well-being or benefit of the individual should be promoted
- the principle of non-maleficence – one ought to do no harm
- the principle of justice – where individuals are considered as equals.

Burkhardt and Nathaniel[13] have added the following three principles:

- veracity – telling the truth

- confidentiality – the protection of a patient's right to privacy[18]
- fidelity – the principle of faithfulness and keeping promises.

Ethical decision making

If nurses are confronted with an ethical issue relating to their patients, they will need to decide how to address it. It could be argued that every decision that a nurse makes about their patients is an ethical one, because there will always be an ethical requirement for the nurse to consider the patient's thoughts, wishes and desires, in order to protect their best interests and maximise their potential for well-being.[7] In order to achieve this, nurses would need an 'objective awareness'[16] where:

- there is a clear understanding of what is beneficial and harmful
- there is no conflict between the nurse's cultural and/or social outlook and the demands of the healthcare setting
- the nurse is a truly human and ethical thinking agent.

This framework of ethical decision making[13] involves a conscious cognitive processing of information and ideas that relates closely to the information-processing model of decision making (*see* Chapter 4).

1 Identification of the pertinent issues relating to the decision or dilemma (e.g. areas of concern, obligation, beliefs and principles).
2 Identification of whose decision it is to make. According to the principle of autonomy, ethical decisions directly relating to the patient should be made by the patient. In some situations the decision will be made by the patient's relatives, although this should be rare (*see* p. 111). In cases where the nurse is not directly involved in the decision, they may act as an information resource or an emotional support.
3 Determination of the moral perspectives of those involved in the decision, and the way that these may influence the decision (e.g. whether they are guided by deontological or utilitarian theory).
4 Determination of the desired outcome, and exclusion of impossible outcomes.
5 Identification of alternative actions, also taking into account legal, professional and economic factors. At this point in the decision-making process the nurse may experience what is known as 'moral distress'. This occurs when they have determined the morally correct course of action, but are unable to pursue it because of limitations imposed by, for example, financial restrictions.[19]
6 Acting on the decision that has been made.

However, ethical dilemmas . . .

Not all decisions will present the nurse with a clearly defined outcome and course of action. They may be confronted with a situation resulting in moral uncertainty, an ethical/moral dilemma or moral distress. *Moral uncertainty* has been described as a situation where the nurse recognises that there is reason for some moral concern, but is not certain either which moral principles apply or what the moral problem might be.[19] For example, suppose that Fred Simms is being cared for at home by his wife, Sarah. Fred regularly comes into Adele's unit for respite care. He seems happy and content, but often appears a little unkempt. To the best of Adele's knowledge, his wife loves him and does her very best to look after him, but Adele feel that Fred's needs are not being completely met.

In a case such as this, Adele would need to be able to answer the following questions:

1 Is Fred able to make decisions relating to how he wants to live?
2 Is Fred able to communicate his decisions?
3 Is Fred being listened to?

There are a number of possibilities here.

1 Fred may be receiving the level of care that he wants.
2 Sarah may be providing care to the best of her ability, but not to the level that she would wish.
3 Sarah may be providing care to the best of her ability, but not to the level that Fred would wish.
4 Sarah may have suggested to Fred that she needs more help, but he has refused to accept this.
5 Both Sarah and Fred would like more help, but none is available.
6 Neither Fred nor Sarah wants any more help, and they are living in the way that they want to live.

Adele is not certain that Fred is not being well cared for, in the way that he wants to be cared for. Fred may never have appeared particularly tidy looking, and this has been his choice, as it may be now. The moral uncertainty here involves issues relating to patient autonomy and choice, and availability of resources. Is Fred still able to make and voice his own choices, and are these being respected? Is it right for nurses to impose their own standards on patients? Is it right for nurses to interfere when patients are living as they choose to live? Is it right for nurses to make patients and their carers feel dissatisfied with healthcare resources when there is no further means of help? Should a nurse always intervene when they suspect that a patient is not being well cared for at home, even if voicing their suspicions could have deep and profound effects on the patient and their carer?

Adele has been presented with a situation for which there is only the possibility of a moral problem, and even that is not clearly defined. Even if she does identify a moral problem, it is possible that the patient, their carers and other nurses may have different moral values and perspectives.

A *moral/ethical dilemma* may present when an individual is confronted with a choice of two ways in which to act, yet there is some inconclusive evidence to suggest both that option A is morally wrong and that option B is morally right. The two courses of action will be mutually inconsistent.[19]

For example, Eric is bed bound, is becoming increasingly frail, and has a very poor prognosis. He has no close family and, in partnership with the nursing staff, doctors have decided that he should not be resuscitated in the event of a cardiac arrest. One afternoon Craig, a junior staff nurse, notices that Eric is unresponsive. He believes that Eric should not simply be left to die, but is fully aware of his condition. Craig is therefore confronted with the choice of two options. It would appear morally right to do everything within his power to save Eric, yet morally wrong to allow him to suffer any longer.

Alternatively, the nurse could be confronted with a situation where they believe that there is moral justification for both performing and not performing an act. For example, Betty has Alzheimer's disease. Some days she is more mentally aware and lucid than others. Her husband Bill died last year, but Betty keeps forgetting this. From time to time she will ask her nurses when Bill is coming to visit, and each time she gets very upset and grief stricken as though it were the first time that she had heard the news. She is having one of her better days today, and seems happy and communicative. She asks Susan when Bill is coming to visit. Susan may consider it morally right to tell Betty the truth about her husband, yet feel that the grief and upset that this would cause her would be morally wrong.[13,15]

A nurse may also be aware of an ethical dilemma when a mentally competent (and therefore legally consensual) patient refuses treatment, or requests that active treatment be discontinued. The nurse will be aware that this may hasten the patient's death, and may find this idea uncomfortable. Assuming that the patient has been fully advised, and has demonstrated understanding of the consequences of their choice, the nurse is both legally and professionally obliged to respect this patient's choice.[9,11,20]

A nurse may experience *moral distress* when they recognise the morally correct course of action, but constraints imposed by the organisation for which they work, or other factors, mean that the pursuit of this action is out of the question.[19] Nurses may experience moral distress, manifested as self-criticism and self-blame, when they are unable to conform to their ideals of 'good' nursing, and may question their own professional competence and knowledge.[21] It is important that nurses accept that there will be constraints on what they do, and can do, yet do not allow this to compromise the standards of care that they aim to provide. Negative expectations can only result in negative outcomes. There is clearly a difference between aiming to provide the best and not quite achieving it, and not expecting to give the best and accomplishing it. Not only will the latter have deleterious effects on patient care, but also it will be unethical, unprofessional and damaging to the nurse's professional self-concept (*see* Chapter 3), which in turn will have a potentially ruinous effect both on patient care and on the nursing profession.

Professional requirements

The humane nature of nursing has already been asserted. Caring is central to nursing, and being able to care is satisfying for nurses.[22] Nurses will experience dissatisfaction if they feel that they are unable to provide effective care. Jean Watson acknowledged the importance of nurses establishing a relationship with their patient, and accepting that they may experience both positive and negative feelings towards that patient.[6,22] Chapter 5 explored some of the ways in which perception can influence nurses' regard of their patients, and the ways in which they involve their patients in decision making.

Stereotypical and prejudicial images of older adults as incapable or incompetent decision makers may distract the nurse from ethical, professional and legal motivations to promote patient autonomy. The importance of healthcare professionals involving their patients in decisions relating to their care has been widely advocated.[2,8] The International Council of Nurses, in its definition of nursing (http://icn.ch/definition/htm), reinforces the importance of nurses working in partnership with their patients regardless of age, culture, environment or status, in the pursuit of health promotion and/or the care of the ill and dying. Specifically, the Nursing and Midwifery Council in the *Code of Professional Conduct*[11] states that nurses, midwives and specialist community public health nurses must respect their patients and clients as individuals:[11]

> You must recognise and respect the role of patients and clients as partners in their care and the contribution they can make to it. This involves identifying their preferences regarding care and respecting these within the limits of professional practice, existing legislation, resources and the goals of the therapeutic relationship.   (p. 5)

If the patient, despite all the nurse's best efforts, is absolutely unable to participate in the decision or discussion, the nurse will have a responsibility to act as their patient's advocate.[17] An advocate has been described as someone who acts on behalf of another, communicating the wishes and desires of an individual who may not be in a position to assert him- or herself.[10] This implies that the nurse would be motivated by the pursuit of the patient's best interests, and in order to achieve this, they must have an awareness of what the patient's interests and beliefs are. This means that even when the patient is not able to make the decision him- or herself, the nurse has an obligation to do everything in their power to find out what the patient's preferences would have been. Moral distress, frustration and anger have been observed in nurses who are unable to fulfil what they perceive to be their role as advocate for vulnerable patients.[23] There is therefore a professional requirement for nurses to take their patient's preferences into account when assessing their needs and planning their care. This professional requirement is reflected both in ethical theory and in the law (p. 5).

Legal requirements

The practice of nurses is bound by the laws of the land, including public laws (governing the operation and provision of health services) and private laws (governing the relationship between organisations and individuals, and providing compensation for victims of malpractice). Civil law covers all public law (except criminal law) and the majority of private law. The premise of civil law is that in the event of some wrongdoing, remedy (usually in the form of a damages payment) may be made to the injured party.[14] Areas of civil law that may be applicable to nurses include applications of tort law where compensation is provided in the event of wrongdoing by one party against another.[14] Examples of torts may include negligence, trespass to property, trespass to the person, false imprisonment, wrongful interference and nuisance.[9] However, there may be occasions when civil law and criminal law intersect – for example, if a nurse has behaved negligently and caused a patient some harm. It may be that the nurse is sued, and pursued only in the civil courts. In other cases, the nurse may also face criminal charges.

The concept of accountability is raised in the Nursing and Midwifery Council *Code of Professional Conduct*:[11]

As a registered nurse, midwife or specialist community public health nurse, you are personally accountable for your practice. In caring for patients and clients, you must:

- respect the patient or client as an individual
- obtain consent before you give any treatment or care
- protect confidential information
- co-operate with others in the team
- maintain your professional knowledge and competence
- be trustworthy
- act to identify and minimise risk to patients and clients.   (p. 3)

This is a professional standard that is supported by law, and Dimond[9] examines the extent to which a nurse can be held responsible for their acts or omissions in law. Reeves and Orford[10] distinguish between a nurse's professional account-ability and responsibilities, suggesting that responsibility can be delegated, but accountability cannot. Accountability comes with experience, but one can be inexperienced and still have responsibilities. One must have authority before being accountable, and allied with accountability is the need to make autono-mous decisions and to be liable for one's actions. Therefore a student nurse may have responsibilities, yet not be accountable, except in circumstances where they are practising without the knowledge and/or consent of their nurse supervisor. Dimond's interpretation focuses on legal responsibility (not taking into account any associated moral or ethical responsibilities), and states that knowledge, including legal knowledge, is a prerequisite of responsibility – 'seen as being liable to be called to account, answerable for, accountable for'[9] (p. 3). Ignorance of the law is not a defence. Dimond[9] defines accountability as being 'concerned with how far the nurse can be held in law to account for her actions' (p. 3), and states that a nurse is accountable in four main areas:

1 the public – criminal law and criminal courts
2 the patient – civil law and civil courts
3 the profession – *Code of Professional Conduct*, Nursing and Midwifery Council
4 the employer – contract of employment, employment tribunal.

The nurse is therefore required to practise within the laws and regulations governing these four areas, and may be held to account if they fail to do so. Although it is expected that the nurse will have an ethical and professional commitment to involving patients in assessments of their needs and in decisions relating to their care, a number of areas of law relate directly to these points. A failure to directly involve the patient could also prove to be illegal.

Although a full examination of the law and its applications is beyond the scope of this book, a number of key areas relating to the assessment of older adults will be examined. These include consent, confidentiality, the Human Rights Act (1998), Do Not Attempt Resuscitation (DNAR) orders, advance directives, and the covert administration of drugs.

Consent

There is recognition in common law of the principle that in all but a few defined circumstances, individuals are protected against non-consensual invasion of their bodily integrity by others.[24] The law states that valid and voluntary consent must be obtained from a mentally competent adult before they are touched. The law does not prescribe the form that consent must take, and it may be actual or implied.[9] The patient must receive information relating to the planned treatment, although there is some contention in law concerning the depth and content of that information.[20] The patient should also demonstrate that they have used their understanding and recall of the information given when making their choice.[9] Consider the following examples.

Expressed consent

Nurse: Mr Smith, I would like to check your pulse just to check that it is safe for me to give you your digoxin this morning.

Mr Smith: Of course, that's fine – it was a bit on the low side yesterday, wasn't it?

Implied consent

Nurse: Mr Smith, I would like to check your pulse just to check that it is safe for me to give you your digoxin this morning.

Mr Smith: (smiling at the nurse, he adjusts his position on the bed and holds up his hand for the nurse to take): Bit on the low side yesterday, wasn't it?

In both cases the patient has indicated that he understands what the nurse is intending to do, and the purpose of the act. There is no evidence that the nurse has coerced the patient or misled him about the reason for checking his pulse rate. The patient has demonstrated that he understands that his pulse needs to be checked before the nurse can safely administer his medication.

Although signing a consent form does provide evidence that a patient has consented to a particular treatment or procedure, it is not proof of consent. If this consent was not obtained, and the nurse actually touched the patient, they would have committed the civil offence of battery. If the patient feared that they would be touched, but the nurse did not actually touch them, this threat would constitute an assault. Furthermore, if the nurse or other healthcare professional failed to provide the patient with adequate or appropriate information when seeking his or her consent, this could be construed as an act of negligence.[20] It is important to remember that not only does the patient have the right to give or withhold their consent, but also they may request the discontinuation of treatment.

Consent by others

At present there is no legitimate capacity for one adult to give proxy consent for healthcare treatment on behalf of another adult. If the patient is judged incapable of providing consent, their family and friends may be consulted in an attempt to find out what the patient's wishes would have been.[25]

However, new legislation in the form of the Mental Capacity Act[26] outlines a statutory framework to support those who lack the capacity to make decisions for themselves. The Act advocates very strongly that wherever possible, individuals should be supported in making their own decisions:

> He [the person making the determination] must, so far as is reasonably practicable, permit and encourage the person to participate, or to improve his ability to participate, as fully as possible in any act done for him and any decision affecting him. (section 4.4)

It does provide some capacity (in specified circumstances) for one adult to give proxy consent for healthcare treatment on behalf of another adult[26] (section 11.7). This legislation will give scope for legal redress against those healthcare professionals who do not involve their patients in the decision-making process.

Exceptions: non-voluntary treatment

Previously, the only exceptions permitted by law were where a patient 'is not in a position to have or to express any views as to his or her management'[24] (p. 220). In cases such as these, treatment was referred to as 'non-voluntary, and applied in situations where the patient's level of consciousness rendered them incapable of consenting, or where their state of mind is such that any consent given would not be valid'.[24] It is likely that implementation of the Mental Capacity Act will result in additional guidelines for practice. But, at present, patients are assumed to be competent unless judged not to be so by a competent practitioner.[11,26] Nurses are currently advised that although they must respect a patient's right to choose, even if that choice may result in them suffering some harm or even death, they should be aware of the procedures should it be necessary to provide care without the patient's consent:[11]

> In emergencies where treatment is necessary to preserve life, you may provide care without consent, if a patient or client is unable to give it, provided you can demonstrate that you are acting in their best interests. (section 3.8, p. 7)

What would constitute best interests? The Nursing and Midwifery Council[11] suggests that acts necessary to preserve the patient's life would be supported (e.g. using suction to clear exudates from the airway of a patient about to choke to death).[24] Acts in cases such as this, and those of alleged negligence, would be subject to judgement relative to what would be judged as reasonable standards by their peers, generally evaluated in law by the application of what has become known as the Bolam test.[27] This arose from direction given to the jury in the Bolam v Friern Hospital Management Committee case in 1957, which declared that a doctor could not be regarded as being in breach of his duty of care 'if he has acted in accordance with a practice accepted as proper by a responsible body of medical men skilled in that particular art'.

In other words, nurses should act in the manner expected of a professional equipped with the same skills, in the same or similar circumstances.

However, there are situations where acting in what the nurse believes to be the patient's best interests would not be permissible – for example, if a patient had made an advance directive (an instruction given by a mentally competent adult outlining their wishes relating to healthcare should circumstances arise where they are no longer able to effectively communicate their wishes; the Mental Capacity Act[26] provides detailed guidelines for healthcare professionals on implementing advance directives).

There is clearly strong legal support for nurses obtaining a patient's consent in most circumstances. However, it has already been suggested in Chapter 6 that in practice this may not happen, with any evidence of cognitive impairment usually being regarded as synonymous with a patient's inability to make informed decisions. For example, patients with dementia are less likely to be involved in decisions relating to DNAR orders than those without dementia.[28] However, this perceived inability is often simply not the case, and research does indicate that patients with some degree of cognitive impairment are able to make informed decisions (*see* Chapter 6). Even if a patient has a fluctuating cognitive state, or varying levels of consciousness, there is a suggestion that any consent given during periods of mental capacity would remain valid during periods of mental incapacity, provided that the issues relating to the consent remain the same.[9]

Looking at Do Not Attempt Resuscitation (DNAR) orders: the legal and ethical implications of involving the patient in decision making

DNAR orders are one aspect of caring for older adults that might cause healthcare professionals to experience ethical dilemmas. On the one hand it is morally wrong to prolong suffering, yet morally right to protect and promote life. Yet it must be acknowledged that in the event of cardiac or respiratory arrest, for some individuals, particularly the terminally ill and the aged reaching the end of their natural life, resuscitation may not be appropriate. There will also be some people who do not wish to be resuscitated in the event of cardiopulmonary arrest, preferring to exercise their right in law to 'die with dignity'.

The British Medical Association, the Royal College of Nursing and the Resuscitation Council (UK)[25] have issued guidance for decisions relating to cardiopulmonary resuscitation which advocates the legal and ethical require-ments to involve patients in decisions relating to their care wherever possible. They recognise that although it is good practice to involve the patient's family and friends in decisions involving the patient, they have no legal right to contribute to those decisions. It is also important that healthcare professionals exercise some caution when considering what relatives tell them about the patient's wishes. In Chapter 6 it was suggested that relatives' perceptions of the patient's preferences may be inaccurate, and it is likely that, in these situations, relatives will be experiencing some emotional distress which could impair their decision-making ability.[29]

The question of whether or not to attempt resuscitation is an emotive one, and some healthcare professionals have voiced concerns about patient involvement in this decision. There have been suggestions that if a patient is very frail and unwell, they may lack the level of consciousness required to consider what may be regarded as rather complex information, and demonstration of such under-standing is a prerequisite of informed consent.[9] Doctors may also find it difficult to present the information in a manner that is easily understood, and to spend the time necessary to support the patient in making this decision.[30] They may also have a paternalistic reluctance to involve the patient in such decision making if they feel that it is not 'practical, sensible or in the patient's best interests',[31] and are wary of presenting patients with information that they fear will distress them, or that will remove any sense of hope for recovery, especially if they feel that resuscitation attempts would be futile in any case. However, there is evidence to suggest that healthcare professionals are not always good at making accurate judgements about the patient's wishes.[30]

There are strong ethical and legal reasons for involving patients in this decision. As with any other aspect of their care, patients have a legal right to either give or withhold their consent, even if their carers sense that such a decision contravenes their ethical principles of preserving life. The potential consequences of ignoring the patient's right to choose are illustrated by the case of Miss B v an NHS Hospital Trust [2002].[32] Miss B was a woman in her forties who suffered a burst blood vessel in her neck that rendered her quadriplegic. She wanted to be able to ask her doctors to turn off the artificial ventilator that was keeping her alive, and Dame Elizabeth Butler-Schloss ruled in her favour, stating that Miss B had the mental capacity necessary to choose to have treatment withdrawn. Furthermore, it was ruled that should anyone attempt to treat Miss B contrary to her will, this would constitute 'unlawful trespass'.

Although it is understandable that nurses and other healthcare professionals are reluctant to put their patients in a position that may distress them, such a paternalistic attitude is ethically, professionally and legally inadmissible. There are ways of approaching emotive subjects that can minimise the patient's distress. For example, with regard to DNAR orders, guidelines suggest that care is taken to present the information as part of the general admission routine, rather than as a suggestion that the patient is likely to experience an imminent cardiopulmonary arrest.[25]

Confidentiality

Ethical, professional and legal obligations require nurses to protect their patient's confidentiality.[20] All patient information should be regarded as confidential if it is acquired during the conduct of professional duties and is not obviously in the public domain. Furthermore, anonymisation of information where it may still be possible to identify the patient will not remove any obligation to maintain confidentiality.[18] Patient autonomy is a valued ethical principle in healthcare. If patients are to be autonomous, then they must have the freedom to decide who has access to confidential information relating to them.[33] Therefore any unauthorised disclosure would be unethical.

Although the interests of the patient should be the primary concern of the nurse, a breach of confidentiality may also result in professional and/or legal sanctions, and nurses need to be aware of their responsibilities and obligations. There are a number of key areas in law which serve to protect patient confidentiality, namely duty of care, confidentiality implied by employment contracts, a duty to keep information passed in confidence confidential, professional requirements, and statutory duties such as the Data Protection Act 1998 and the Human Rights Act (Article 8).[9]

However, the disclosure of confidential information may be permissible in a limited number of exceptional circumstances, listed below, although nurses should seek advice before disclosing information on this or any other basis.[18]

1 If the patient has given their informed consent for the information to be released. This consent is limited to specific pieces of information, and can only be given if the patient has an understanding of who is to receive the

information, the purpose of the disclosure and the possible outcomes of the disclosure. If the patient is incapable of giving their consent, any disclosure must only be made if it is in the patient's best interests.

2 If the law (either court order or under statute) orders disclosure – for example, the Public Health Control of Diseases Act 1984 or the Prevention of Terrorism Act. The police and the courts have no statutory power to seize confidential patient information, unless it is to prevent the records from being destroyed (under the Police and Criminal Evidence Act 1984). Court orders may be made to release clinical records in the case of litigation.

3 When a disclosure of information is in the public interest – for example, if there is a real risk of serious public harm or crime.

The Nursing and Midwifery Council[11] recommends that nurses ensure that patients are aware that information relating to them may be shared with other professionals involved in their care, as it would be impractical to obtain consent every time there is a need to communicate about the patient. It also suggests that nurses find out their patients' wishes with regard to communication of information to their family and friends. Nurses may find that they have breached confidentiality regulations if they have discussed care with the relatives without the patient's consent. They should not assume that because a patient is confused or has impaired communication, they wish their affairs to be discussed with their family. The Nursing and Midwifery Council offers a professional advice service that can help nurses with issues relating to confidentiality. It can be accessed via their website (www.nmc-uk.org).

The Human Rights Act (1998)[34]

The International Council of Nursing[35] has advocated the role of nurses in promoting and protecting the human rights of their patients:

> Human rights in healthcare involve both recipients and providers. . . .
> This right includes the right to choose or decline care, including the right to accept or refuse treatment or nourishment; informed consent; confidentiality, and dignity, including the right to die with dignity.

Existing laws, professional codes and ethical principles protected many of these rights (e.g. consent).[36] However, from October 2000, the Human Rights Act 1998 brought the rights and freedoms identified by the European Convention on Human Rights into the realm of UK law. Prior to that, UK citizens were required to seek redress through the European Court of Human Rights in Strasbourg – an often lengthy process.

An individual's fundamental rights are outlined in the Articles of Schedule 1 of the Act. The Human Rights Act (1998) can be downloaded from http://hmso.gov.uk/acts/acts1998/80042, and there is a legal obligation for individuals working with public authorities to protect these rights. Although implementation of the Act is still relatively new, and open to some interpretation in law, an examination of some of the Articles will show that the Act should lend additional support to many of the reasons already advocated for involving patients in assessments and decisions relating to their care.

Article 2 – Right to Life

> Everyone's right to life shall be protected by law.

Life is precious, and healthcare professionals have an obligation to work to safeguard life.

Article 3 – Prohibition of Torture

> No one shall be subjected to torture or to inhuman or degrading treatment or punishment.

It could be judged that any care imposed on a patient that does not address their own wishes and preferences does not take account of their autonomy and right to choose, and could therefore be construed as inhuman or degrading.

Article 8 – Right to Respect for Private and Family Life

> Everyone has the right to respect for his private and family life, his home and his correspondence.

Patients have a right to their privacy, to live as they choose. If patients are not truly involved in an assessment, how will this be facilitated?

Article 9 – Freedom of Thought, Conscience and Religion

> Everyone has the right to freedom of thought, conscience and religion.

Again, every patient has the right to live their life according to their personal choices, beliefs and principles.

Article 10 – Freedom of Expression

> Everyone has the right to freedom of expression. This right shall include freedom to hold opinions and to receive and impart ideas without interference by public authority and regardless of frontiers.

Healthcare professionals must respect their patients' right to their own views and opinions regarding the way they live and their approaches to healthcare.

Article 12 – Right to Marry

> Men and women of marriageable age have the right to marry and found a family.

Older patients have a right to pursue and protect their needs for companionship and partnership.

Article 14 – Prohibition of Discrimination

> The enjoyment of the rights and freedoms set forth in this Convention shall be secured without discrimination on any ground such as sex, race, colour, language, religion, political or other opinion, national or social origin, association with a national minority, property, birth or other status.

Although discrimination on the basis of age is not specifically mentioned, it may be included by implication in the use of the phrase 'such as'.

The worst-case scenario – abuse of vulnerable older adults: what protection is there in law?

Action on Elder Abuse[37] defines elder abuse as:

> A single or repeated act or lack of appropriate action, occurring within any relationship where there is an expectation of trust, which causes harm or distress to an older patient.

Elder abuse can be physical (beating, pinching, over-sedation, giving the incorrect medication, dressing the patient inappropriately for the climate conditions), psychological (humiliating, ignoring, swearing, 'talking over'), financial (stealing, extorting of funds), sexual (inappropriate touching, exposure, any sexual contact without consent) or neglect by caregivers (not assisting with hygiene needs, depriving of food, depriving of fluids, leaving the patient in soiled clothing). Any act by a person in a position of power that is detrimental to the humanity of an older person may constitute an act of elder abuse.[37]

What legal protection is there for vulnerable older adults?

1 The Human Rights Act (1998)[34] infers some protection of the rights of vulnerable older adults.
2 The Mental Capacity Act (2005)[26] introduces some statutory provision for legislation against those in a position of power who neglect or ill-treat adults with an impaired capacity to make decisions for themselves.
3 The Protection of Vulnerable Adults list introduced by the Department of Health in 2004[38] means that care workers who have either harmed or put at risk of harm a vulnerable older adult will be prohibited from caring (in a place of work) for vulnerable older adults in the future. However, at the time of writing this scheme is limited to care workers employed by registered providers of care homes and domiciliary care agencies, including those supplied by employment agencies.
4 Civil or criminal proceedings against the abuser, but this is often difficult because the abused person may be unwilling or unable to make a complaint.[37]
5 Professional misconduct procedures.

The Nursing and Midwifery Council has published guidelines advising on the practitioner–client relationship and the prevention of abuse. This can be accessed via their website (www.nmc-uk.org).

In summary

This chapter has explored ethical, professional and legal factors relating to decision making and the nurse caring for older patients. There is a strong consensus that in all but exceptional cases (perhaps if the patient is comatose or at the very end stage of their life and unable to communicate), the nurse should make every endeavour to involve their patient in decision making. This will be inherent to the assessment process, and the nurse will need to find out the patient's preferences and wishes.

The nurse should not make assumptions about their patient's decision-making ability, and should not without very good reason defer to relatives and informal carers for patient information. If nurses fail to respect their patient's right to involvement, they will be acting unethically, unprofessionally and illegally.

Key points

- Nurses must always act in the patient's best interests.
- Nurses may be required to make some ethically difficult decisions.
- Regardless of how they may appear, in most circumstances the patient can and should be involved in decisions relating to their care.
- If it has been determined by a suitably qualified practitioner that a patient is incapable of participating in the decision-making process, the nurse should endeavour to find out what the patient's preferences would have been.
- However, nurses must be careful not to breach their patient's right to confidentiality.
- In most circumstances the patient's informed consent must be obtained before the nurse releases confidential information relating to them.
- Relatives and friends should not be approached for information if the patient is capable of providing that information him- or herself.
- In most circumstances the patient's informed consent must be obtained before the nurse performs any kind of care procedure on them.
- At present, no adult can give consent on behalf of another adult. In circumstances where a doctor regards a patient as incompetent to make a decision, they must act in the patient's best interests.

References

1 Burnard P (1997) Why care? Ethical and spiritual issues in caring nursing. In: G Bryckczynska (ed.) *Caring. The compassion and wisdom of nursing.* Edward Arnold, London.
2 Department of Health (2001) *The Essence of Care.* The Stationery Office, London.
3 Walsh K and Kowanko I (2002) Nurses' and patients' perceptions of dignity. *Int J Nurs Pract.* **8:** 143–51.
4 Ghaye T, Gillespie D and Lilleyman S (2000) *Empowerment Through Reflection: the narratives of healthcare professionals.* Quay Books, Mark Allen Publishing Ltd, Dinton.
5 Rodwell CM (1996) An analysis of the concept of empowerment. *J Adv Nurs.* **21:** 682–9.
6 Taylor HJ (2000) A caring moment with Margaret. In: T Ghaye and S Lilleyman (eds) *Caring Moments: the discourse of reflective practice.* Quay Books, Mark Allen Publishing Ltd, Dinton.
7 Singleton J and McLaren S (1995) *Ethical Foundations of Healthcare.* Mosby, London.
8 Department of Health (2000) *The NHS Plan: a plan for investment, a plan for reform.* The Stationery Office, London.
9 Dimond B (2005) *Legal Aspects of Nursing* (4e). Pearson Longman, Harlow.

10 Reeves M and Orford J (2002) *Fundamental Aspects of Legal, Ethical and Professional Issues in Nursing.* Quay Books, Mark Allen Publishing Ltd, Dinton.

11 Nursing and Midwifery Council (2004) *The NMC Code of Professional Conduct: standards for conduct, performance and ethics.* Nursing and Midwifery Council, London.

12 Tschudin V (1994) *Ethics: conflicts of interest.* Scutari Press, London.

13 Burkhardt MA and Nathaniel AK (2002) *Ethics and Issues in Contemporary Nursing* (2e). Delmar: Thompson Learning Ltd, Clifton Park, NY.

14 Hendrick J (2000) *Law and Ethics in Nursing and Healthcare.* Stanley Thornes, Cheltenham.

15 Beauchamp TL and Childress JF (1994) *Principles of Biomedical Ethics* (4e). Oxford University Press, Oxford.

16 Husted GL and Husted JH (1995) *Ethical Decision Making in Nursing.* Mosby, St Louis, MO.

17 Burnard P and Chapman C (2000) *Professional and Ethical Issues In Nursing* (3e). Baillière Tindall, London.

18 Dolan B (2004) Medical records: disclosing confidential clinical information. *Psychiatr Bull.* **28:** 53–6.

19 Jameton A (1984). *Nursing Practice: the ethical issues.* Prentice Hall, Englewood Cliffs, NJ.

20 Montgomery J (1997) *Healthcare Law.* Oxford University Press, New York.

21 Kelly B (1998) Preserving moral integrity: a follow-up study with new graduate nurses. *J Adv Nurs.* **28:** 1134–45.

22 Watson J (1989) Philosophy and science of caring. In: A Marriner-Tomey (ed.) *Nursing Theorists and Their Work.* Mosby, St Louis, MO.

23 Sundin-Huard D and Fahy K (1999) Moral distress, advocacy and burnout: theorizing the relationships. *Int J Nurs Pract.* **5:** 8–13.

24 Mason JK and McCall Smith RA (1994) *Law and Medical Ethics.* Butterworth and Co. Publishers, London.

25 British Medical Association, Resuscitation Council (UK) and Royal College of Nursing (2001) *Decisions Relating to Cardio-Pulmonary Resuscitation.* Ethics Department, British Medical Association, London.

26 Mental Capacity Act (2005) Elizabeth II. Chapter 9. www.opsi.gov.uk/acts/acts2005/50009--a.htm (accessed 30/6/05).

27 *Bolam v. Friern Barnet HMC* [1957] 2 All ER 118.

28 Haydar ZR *et al.* (2004) Differences in end-of life preferences between congestive heart failure and dementia in a medical house calls programme. *J Am Geriatr Soc.* **52:** 736–40.

29 Forbes S, Bern-Klu M and Gessert C (2000) End-of-life decision making for nursing home residents with dementia. *J Nurs Scholarship.* **32:** 251–8.

30 Higginson IJ (2003) Doctors should not discuss resuscitation with terminally ill patients. *BMJ.* **327:** 615–15.

31 Manistry C and Waxman J (2003) Doctors should not discuss resuscitation with terminally ill patients. *BMJ.* **327:** 614–15.

32 *Miss B v an NHS Hospital Trust* [2002] 1 FLR 1090 Butler-Schloss. P.

33 O'Brien J and Chantler C (2003) Confidentiality and the duties of care. *J Med Ethics.* **29:** 36–40.

34 Human Rights Act (1998). Chapter 42.

35 International Council of Nursing (1998) *Position Statement: nurses and human rights*; www.icn.ch/pshumrights.htm (accessed 15/02/05).

36 McHale J and Gallagher A (2003) *Nursing and Human Rights.* Butterworth-Heinemann, Oxford.

37 *Action on Elder Abuse*; www.elderabuse.org.uk/Mainpages/Questions.htm (accessed 15/10/04).

38 Department of Health (2004) *Protection of Vulnerable Adults Scheme.* The Stationery Office, London.

Index